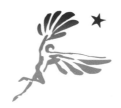

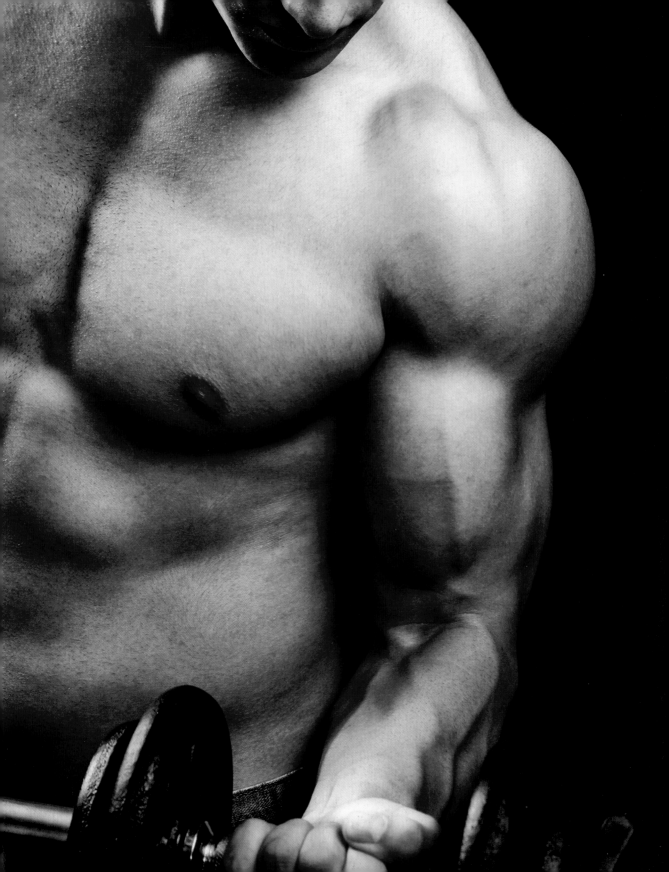

THE *BODYBUILDING*.com®

GUIDE TO

YOUR BEST BODY

**THE REVOLUTIONARY 12-WEEK PLAN TO TRANSFORM
YOUR BODY AND STAY FIT FOREVER**

KRIS GETHIN

Editor at Large of Bodybuilding.com

with Gretchen Lees

A TOUCHSTONE BOOK

Published by Simon & Schuster

New York   London   Toronto   Sydney   New Delhi

Touchstone
A Division of Simon & Schuster, Inc.
1230 Avenue of the Americas
New York, NY 10020

Copyright © 2011 by Bodybuilding.com, LLC

Previously published under the title *Body by Design*

First Touchstone trade paperback edition December 2012

TOUCHSTONE and colophon are registered trademarks of Simon & Schuster, Inc.

For information about special discounts for bulk purchases, please contact Simon & Schuster Special Sales at 1-866-506-1949 or business@simonandschuster.com.

The Simon & Schuster Speakers Bureau can bring authors to your live event. For more information or to book an event contact the Simon & Schuster Speakers Bureau at 1-866-248-3049 or visit our website at www.simonspeakers.com.

Designed by Ruth Lee-Mui

Manufactured in the United States of America

10 9 8 7 6 5 4 3 2 1

The Library of Congress has cataloged the hardcover edition as follows:
Gethin, Kris.
   Body by design / by Kris Gethin.
      p. cm.
   "A Touchstone book."
   Includes index.
   1. Weight training. 2. Bodybuilding—Training. 3. Physical fitness. I. Title.
   GV545.5.G47 2011
   613.7'13—dc22
                                          2010038726

ISBN 978-1-4516-0217-3
ISBN 978-1-4516-0631-3 (pbk)
ISBN 978-1-4516-0614-0 (ebook)

DEDICATION

I dedicate this book to the most influential people who have shaped my life physically, mentally, and spiritually. My wife, best friend, and the air that I breathe, Marika, you are the center of my purpose. I have always learned more by observing people rather than asking questions, and for that I thank the community of BodySpace for allowing me to witness your friendship, support, and the transformation of your lives—it has helped me evolve so I can now virally help others.

CONTENTS

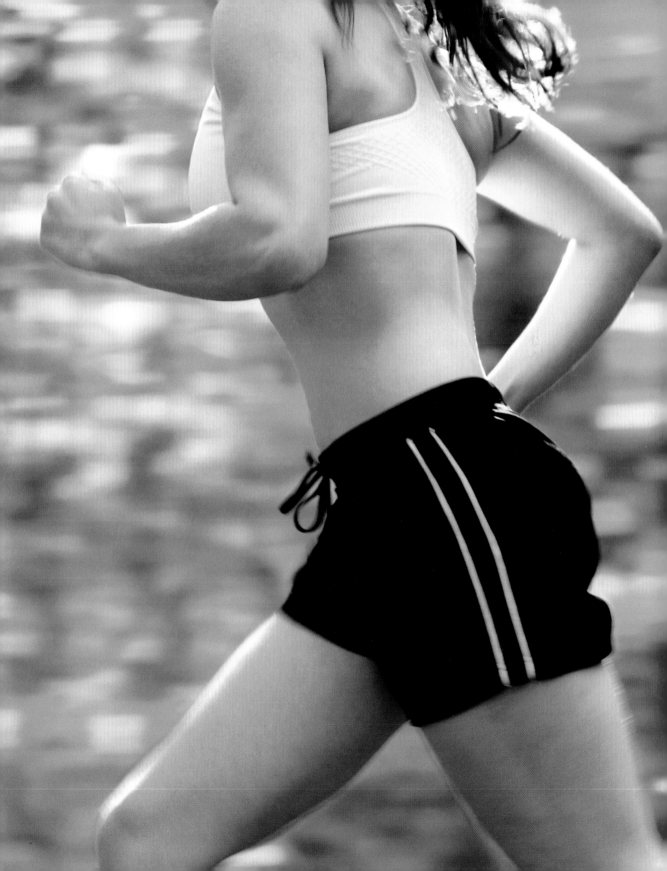

FOREWORD by Jamie Eason

Ask just about anyone for the key to improved health and wellness and the likely answer would be: a healthy diet and exercise routine. While it seems that we are all well aware of the benefits, sticking to a program with any sort of real consistency is where many repeatedly fall short. Take me for example: There have been countless times that I would promise myself that I would start eating right and exercising, yet come Monday, I would rationalize that I was too busy to make it to the gym and my idea of eating right often simply meant choosing the lesser of two evils. The only thing routine about my routine was its tendency to fail.

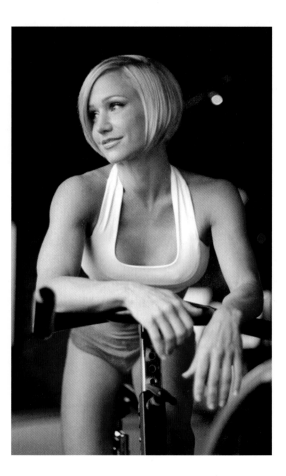

It was not until a diagnosis of early stage breast cancer that I found the resolve to really stick with making healthier choices and getting regular exercise. Yet, even with a catalyst as serious as cancer, I still found sticking to a routine and staying motivated very challenging. Not only did I have my own willpower to contend with but outside influences, such as the people around me who profoundly influenced me as well. After many failed attempts to maintain my healthy habits while still engaging in my usual social behaviors of nights out with friends and eating out with family, I knew something had to give. I knew that I would never assimilate to a healthier lifestyle as long as I was surrounded by the wrong influences, but where could I find the right influences? The answer was the Internet and more specifically, BodySpace.

As you turn the page and discover *The Bodybuilding.com Guide to Your Best Body* you'll find, just as I did, how connecting with like-minded people from all walks of life can help you reach your goals. Contained within these pages, my friend and author Kris Gethin, will present you with some of the most compelling and inspirational stories of people who have used the site to turn tragedy into triumph or who simply found the resolve to make last-

ing change. With over a half million people on BodySpace, Kris Gethin and I have witnessed firsthand the true power of connecting to the right social influences. We have watched people shed negative influences, replacing them with new positive ones and we have witnessed how being transparent and open with goals can rally support and accountability from those around you. At any given moment someone can log onto BodySpace to find help or encouragement and that sort of support system has proven to be invaluable for making progress and reaching goals.

Now it's your turn to discover the incredible support that a positive social network can lend to the success of your personal fitness goals. *The Bodybuilding.com Guide to Your Best Body* will introduce you to the same fitness and motivation principles that have guided hundreds of thousands of people to incredible results. This book finally answers the question of how to stay motivated. Let Kris guide you to ultimate success with a sound eating and exercise plan and an even stronger motivational foundation. All you must do is take the first step and turn the page.

—Jamie Eason

TRANSFORMATION Nation

I want to make something clear right up front: **this book is not about me, it's about *you*.** It's not about the latest diet or exercise fad that's "guaranteed to get you fit fast." (In case you haven't figured this out on your own: those fads don't work.) It doesn't stand a chance of landing on an infomercial or finding its way to the drugstore aisle. I promise you, you will find no gimmicks here. What you will find is a program that was created by people just like you, for people just like you. People who thought they didn't have enough time or energy to get fit, people dealing with illness or disability, some who are managing relationships, children, and busy careers; others who like to go to parties and clubs and still want to look great on the beach; and still others who were morbidly obese or dangerously thin. You name the obstacle, condition, or circumstance, and I can tell you that this program didn't just help them to overcome it but helped them discover the drive to thrive despite all their excuses not to do so. I call it the Body by Design plan.

The Bodybuilding.com Guide to Your Best Body isn't just a book; it's a movement. A movement is the shared and organized pursuit of a common goal, and as editor in chief of the world's leading fitness Web site, Bodybuilding .com, I have seen hundreds of thousands of people pursue the common goal of achieving lasting health and fitness. By tapping into the wellspring of connection, information, and motivation available within the community on our site, called BodySpace, I have seen many of them not only fulfill this goal but experience what can only be called a life transformation. You'll hear me refer to BodySpace a lot over the course of this book. BodySpace has created a virtual meeting ground for nearly two million people, who have discovered there the tools and, more important, the team they need to make health a way of life.

In this book you will discover many of these transformational stories and the program that brought this reinvention process to life. I've packaged everything I've learned from people just like you and brought the movement to the pages you hold in your hands. Consider this your official invitation to join—to become a part of what I refer to as Transformation Nation. This is not an exclusive club; it doesn't require a membership card or have any prerequisites. All it takes is a simple statement from you: *I'm ready*.

MY STORY

You're probably wondering who I am. My name is Kris Gethin, and first and foremost, I am a person who lives and breathes fitness. I take pride in my health, and I am driven to keep my body in top form because it is the hub from which all other parts of life extend. I am here because my role at Bodybuilding.com has given me inside access to truly incredible people who have inspired me and who continue to redefine the limits of human possibility—I am here as their ambassador and as the messenger who comes bearing the blueprint for personal change. Before we get to their stories, though, I want to tell you a little about my own transformation.

I was born and raised in Wales in the United Kingdom. I lived on a farm and learned early on about the value of a strong work ethic (and the equally important value of a strong back, arms, and legs). I tried lifting weights here and there, but in my early teenage years what I really fell in love with was motocross (for the uninitiated, it's like cross-country motorcycle racing). I loved the sport so much that I did just about everything I could to keep my weight down for it, because the lighter you are, the faster you go. I was into riding BMX bikes, running, cardio, and swimming. I have asthma, which held me back a lot, but it didn't stop me from doing what I loved. It was around that time that I started buying all the bodybuilding magazines I could get my hands on. I would flip through the pages and stare at the pictures in disbelief—I looked at those guys as real-life superheroes. I was so inspired by their level of fitness that it helped me work harder on my own body.

A few years down the road my love for extreme sports led me to a group of extreme athletes. I discovered that they were intense people in every way—pushing the limits on the racecourse as well as in the bars and on the party circuit. Before I knew it my social network had shaped me into a different person with different priorities from the ones I had always had. I knew it was time for a change, and I also knew that I had to get out of my social group to make the change transformational and lasting. This triggered a new direction for me, and I went back to school to study international health and sports therapy, which eventually led to my touring the world as a health and fitness expert on a cruise line.

I spent years working with individuals and small groups as a personal trainer and even ran my own gym for a while. I loved connecting with people and motivating them toward their fitness goals, but I wanted to find a vehicle for reaching and connecting with more peo-

ple. That's when I started writing and photographing images for fitness magazines; I figured this way my work could connect with thousands of people

BEFORE

AFTER

instead of just a few at a time. I began interacting with more people in the fitness world, and it was a thrill to discover that my research, knowledge, and experience were reaching a growing number of people on a consistent basis. I moved to Los Angeles, California, because I figured it would give me the chance to bump shoulders with some of the biggest names in fitness. But subconsciously I was still searching for the right group culture fit—and I didn't find it until I made my way to Bodybuilding.com.

The best part of the discovery was not just that my work ethic and goals had found their perfect match, but that within the site there existed BodySpace, a community filled with some of the most solid, driven, and motivating people I would ever meet; I discovered there what I had been missing in Wales and Los Angeles: a steady and inspirational group of like-minded people who would check out my work, look to me for knowledge, *and* fuel my own drive to be at the top of my game. It's been a win-win relationship ever since.

I'm sure you have a story similar to my own—one filled with experiences that shaped your future as they were filtered through the influence of your friends, family, or other social group. For me, the major turning points in my life were those that involved these outside influences—leaving my group of friends in Wales probably saved my life, just as discovering the BodySpace community helped change my life from good to great. The people who surround us—our friends, families, classmates, coworkers, neighbors, and even the person driving in the car next to us—can greatly influence our choices and behaviors on a large or incredibly small level. These influences are really the foundation from which all transformational change can happen.

Now that you know a little about my story, I'd like you to start writing the next, better chapter of your own life. Your journey will begin from the inside out, starting with the thoughts in your head and working its way to the muscles in your body and the food on your plate. I will guide you down the most powerful and proven path to change, which will be supplemented by the motivational discoveries and success stories of the BodySpace community members who have paved the way for you. Be sure too to check out the Instant Inspiration blurbs throughout the book for quick bursts of motivation! They include each person's first name and BodySpace username, should you wish to find their full profile online at www.bodyspace.com.

Welcome to Body by Design, the fitness movement that's going to change your life.

> Your journey will begin from the inside out, starting with the thoughts in your head and working its way to the muscles in your body and the food on your plate.

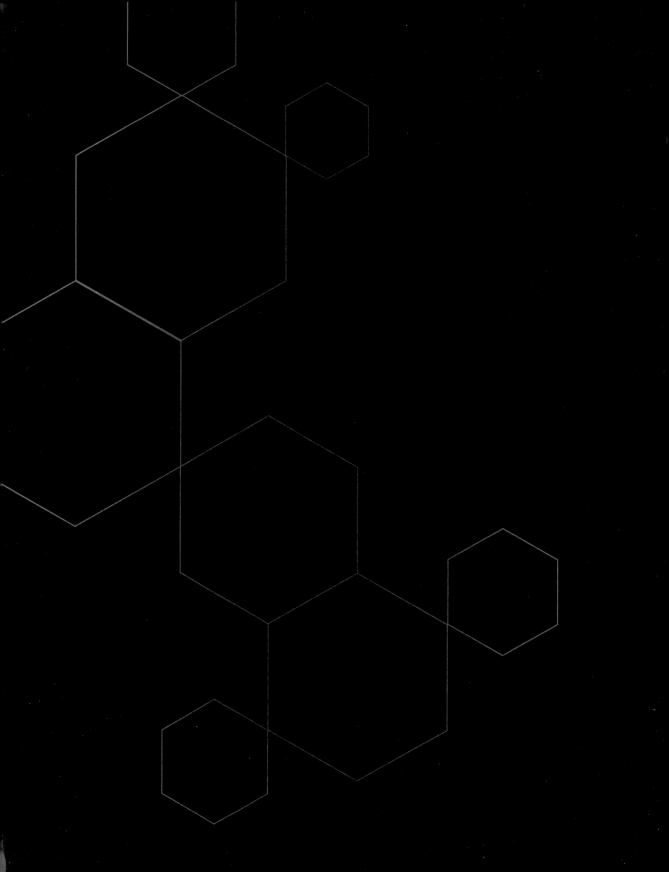

THE *BODYBUILDING*.com®

GUIDE TO

YOUR BEST BODY

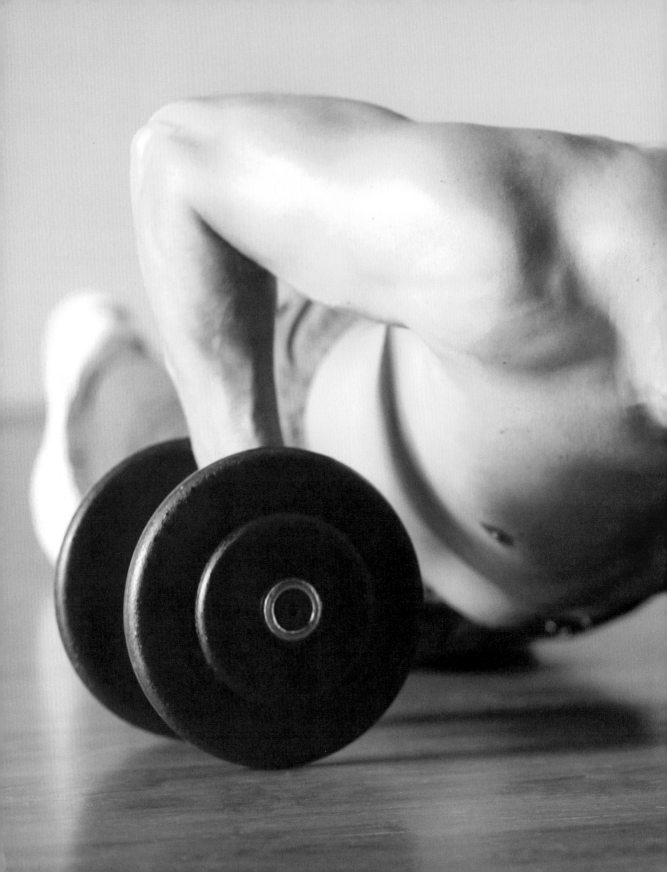

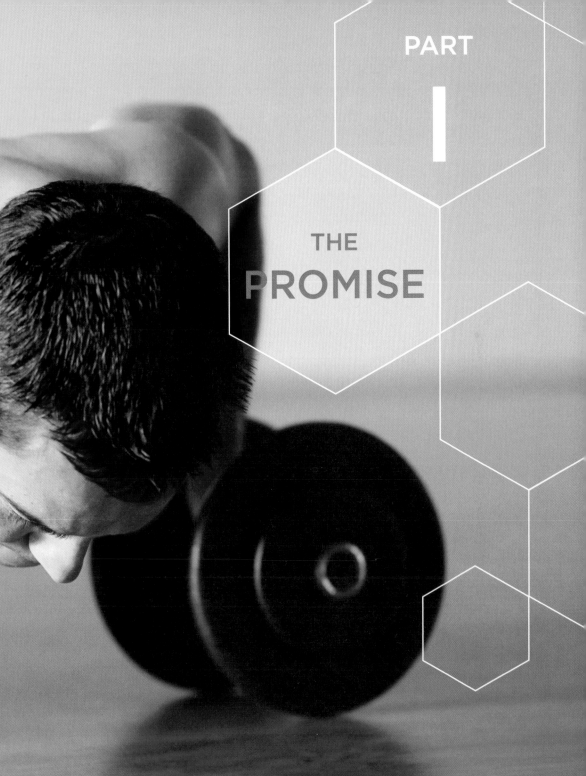

THE
PROMISE

CHAPTER 1

Are You Ready to CHANGE Your Life?

What if I told you that ultimate fitness success does not come from doing the right number of reps, burning the correct number of calories, or eating the perfect amount of protein? That groundbreaking research in motivational science has revealed that true fitness comes instead from **connecting to a proven system of motivational support?**

You might think it just another false pledge delivered to you from the world of health and fitness, a story that will lead you down the same road of unfulfilled promises and disappointing results. If that's the case, I want to tell you another story.

THE CAPTAIN'S STORY

Several years ago, I met a man who was so tormented by phantom pain after losing a leg that he was pumping himself full of morphine just to make life bearable. His doctor said his pain was so severe that even the strongest medications couldn't stand up to it for long. Feeling helpless, this man self-medicated his depression and post-traumatic stress disorder with pounds of junk food and at least three bottles of wine a night. Losing his leg challenged his manhood and took him to the darkest space he had ever known—he wanted to end his life. He went as far as setting a plan into motion, lining the walls of a room in his house with clear plastic so his wife wouldn't have to have to clean up a big mess after the deed was done.

What happened next to this man, whom I will call "Captain Ahab" (his real name is Errol, but I think his chosen nickname really captures his fighting spirit), is an astounding example of human power and resilience. His wife, who had witnessed him in devastating pain day in and day out, knew he had the strength to overcome it. She was suffering from lupus and fibromyalgia and suggested they fight back against the pain by taking control of their bodies. She proposed that they enter a fitness challenge.

They started strength training together, and gradually Captain Ahab began to see his body change. Miraculously, lifting weights delivered a relief from his phantom leg pain—it literally made it go away for hours at a time—giving him a truly priceless gift. This man made a lasting comeback from the brink by transforming himself through fitness, not just because he discovered strength training and changed his *body* but because he anchored this process to an unshakable network of support and changed his *life*.

He found this network of support when he joined BodySpace. Captain Ahab's commitment to fitness went from transitional to transformational because by creating a profile and sharing his goals there, he turned a private commitment into a public one. He also discovered there a solid chain of inspiration and motivation fueled by members' feedback and friendly guidance.

Captain Ahab now finds himself motivated not by future goals or results but by other people. He reads stories about others' success and is fueled by their achievements and their constant stream of inspirational comments and messages. This motivation is regenerated when they say that *he's* inspired *them*—their deep appreciation for his recovery and transformation pushes him even further.

The story of Captain Ahab is true, and it's only one of the many transformations I've witnessed when people connect to a structured system of motivational support and make a few critical

A LITTLE MORE ABOUT BodySpace™ SOCIAL FITNESS NETWORK

If you haven't heard about BodySpace, don't worry—it's not something you have to buy in order for this program to work for you. It's a no-cost online community filled with people (including me) who are pursuing various health and fitness goals and want to connect with others doing the same. Bodyspace is a completely free Web site (like Facebook or other social networking sites) that lets users create a customized profile that can include everything from progress pictures to accomplishments, goals, and much more.

Members connect with other members by sharing messages and comments with one another, creating a constant exchange of information and motivation. They also advance their own fitness programs through these connections and create BodyGroups, which are groups of members who've discovered matching goals or similar backgrounds or age. To create your own profile, visit www.bodyspace.com.

changes to their diet and fitness regime. This revolutionary approach, which is at the core of the Body by Design program, extends and breathes new life into the old-school methods of goal pursuit. It's what happens when you marry tangible rewards (a great body being just one of them) to a deeper sense of fulfillment.

Captain Ahab's story (read more about him and his wife on pages 13–16), which continues to amaze me, is unique, but his experience of personal transformation isn't; nor is it surprising once you understand the system that set him up for success. He changed his life by accessing a practical toolbox for fitness success and supporting the elements in it with an immense, dependable community of support. Friends and virtual neighbors he'd never known existed came out to help him rebuild his life—and now he's ready to return the favor.

"I am no longer broken; I feel as though I have been reborn. I have never been more focused in my life. My real goal is to assist people in overcoming the obstacles that are stopping them from achieving the weight loss they desire and reaching their fitness goals."

WHAT ARE YOUR FITNESS ROADBLOCKS?

When you consider someone like Captain Ahab, you might think about the obstacles that have gotten in your way—the ones that have stopped you from sticking to your commitments to exercise more and eat better. The most common perceived obstacles are lack of time, fear of trying something new or difficult, and situational factors such as a lack of family support or access to a gym. As you may recall,

I myself struggled with how to get out of an enticing community of hard-partying friends to pursue my true passions of health and fitness. When you really think about it, none of those roadblocks sounds too tough to overcome when compared to something like Captain Ahab's phantom leg pain, but they are real obstacles and excuses that people use every day to keep them from pursuing or fulfilling a fitness goal.

Here's what I want you to understand: **every single reason or excuse can be faced head-on and obliterated when you focus on** *motivation* **as the single greatest challenge in achieving your fitness goals.** The best thing is that motivation is *built into you*—and when you tap into the right system of support, it's activated automatically. Until you discover that system, you will continue to see obstacles as walls, but if you're ready to break them down, I am ready to show you how you can do it.

When you discover this cutting-edge, science-supported motivational system, you will learn how to create a behavior change that promises long-lasting, not short-term, results. You will enhance and enrich your life by adding things to it instead of subtracting—no more focusing on shortsighted negative goals, such as *cutting out* calories, *losing* weight, *banishing* your belly. Instead, you will focus on *adding* more muscle, *amplifying* your support base, and *maximizing* your motivational foundation. Finally, you will stop feeling limited by your personal surroundings and form a plan to regain control of your life. No matter where

you are in life, you have at least some power to shape your surroundings and circumstances. But before I introduce you to this system in Chapter 2, I want to stamp out a few pervasive misunderstandings about achieving fitness goals—think of this as knocking down those old walls so you can build a better, stronger foundation for success.

WHY ARE WE STILL STRUGGLING WITH OUR WEIGHT?

Do a quick search online for the phrase "get six-pack abs," and you will get more than a million results; try "weight loss," and you will get more than *ninety-nine million* results. Or let's say you're looking for a book that will show you the way to ideal health and fitness—there were more than 25,000 books published in the field in the last two years alone!

Considering all the information available to us, would you guess that we are a fit, healthy, energized population? If you said "yes," you must live in the one state in this country that has an overweight or obese percentage below 20 percent (Colorado). For the rest of us the answer would be a flabby, unhealthy, dripping-in-fat "no." In fact, as you might have heard, we are in the midst of an obesity epidemic that is producing a scary ripple effect, with our health-care system crippled by conditions and diseases related to obesity, our productivity levels sinking to ever-lower levels, and our children headed for the alarming distinction of being the first generation in the industrial world to have a shorter life span than their parents. Not surprisingly, we're not happy either, with depression, feelings of isolation, and dissatisfaction on the rise. In short, despite our awareness and best intentions, we continue to be stuck in big trouble.

The obvious question here would be: if we have more information on diet and fitness than ever before, why can't we achieve the goal of living healthy, happy, and fulfilled lives? The seemingly obvious answer is that none of those millions of diet and fitness programs work—we simply haven't found the magic formula yet.

What if I told you that the exact opposite is true: that *every single one* of those programs work; that each one contains at the minimum one invaluable kernel of advice that can help you lose weight, get in shape, build muscle, or any combination of the three? This epidemic is not about a lack of information; it's about a lack of motivation.

I'm not talking about motivation of the superficial clichéd variety, the type that's all talk and no action. I'm referring to a proven, permanent structure of motivational support based on strength in numbers, not just the power of one. You are going to discover the power to change your body and your life for the better and for good—with a little help from your friends.

I fully expect some of you to be a bit rankled by the suggestion that you aren't motivated. Believe me, I'm an independent, driven guy, and I used to feel that all the fuel I needed could come from my own solid tank of motivation. I never played team sports or truly understood what it meant to have a network of support. That was until I grew tired of unfulfilled commitments and inconsistent results; it was then that I discovered a group of people with shared goals who pushed me to higher and greater peaks of achievement—places I could never have gone on my own. It's easy to stick to your patterns, even if they make you unhappy and the end result is always the same. What's challenging is to open up your life to new and limitless potential. But trust me, once you do you will never look back.

IT'S TIME TO MAKE A LASTING CHANGE

You've picked up this book because you're ready for a change. Maybe you're tired of not realizing your peak potential, of continually falling short of your goals because you run out of personal steam and lack a system of accountability to pick you back up. Or perhaps you have vowed to not be one of the millions of people who pass on poor health habits to their kids. Or it may be that you never, ever again want to feel embarrassed to take off your shirt at the beach or pool. If you're like Tiffany Forni, now a fitness evangelist, you have more than 100 pounds to lose and you need the community and fitness guidance to help you get started *and* to keep you going all the way to your goal (read her full story on page 28). Or, like thousands of others who've used the tools I share in the Body by Design program, you want to use strength training to maximize your performance in other sports and activities.

INSTANT INSPIRATION

"The transformations on BodySpace keep me motivated and make me want to be an example of health for my daughter. I want her to grow up respecting and loving her body."
—Kassandre*Making_A_Change

Whatever goal or goals you bring to the table, I will help you refine your focus and stop chasing what amounts to nothing more than a mirage of change. You want more than a temporary change with a termination date like all the other fitness books or programs you've tried—you want a permanent change, a lifestyle overhaul that will put you once and for all on the right track to health and fitness. While those other plans might work for the short term (because that's as long as they're intended to work), they fail to provide a platform for indestructible commitment and long-lasting success. They fail because their platform overlooks and undervalues the single greatest factor in achieving your goals and instead places emphasis on the information—information that *could* work if only you had the motivation to stick with it.

I can say this to you because I've seen it happen over and over again: perfectly determined people never achieving their goals because they aren't taught how to tap into their motivation, the most profound and infinite driver of success. They may commit to a program for two days or two weeks, but if they hit a plateau or fall short on personal motivation, as inevitably happens, they fail. Remember: anyone can get his hands on the *information* they need for accomplishing their fitness goals. My 60-year-old dad living in the Welsh countryside can do a quick search online and find out what he needs to eat and the workouts he needs to do to get into great shape. It's not a secret or hidden formula. The problem is that getting only the information is like getting a brand-new sports car without being handed the keys—all that power and potential remain just a cold, useless hunk of steel without the keys. When you add in the essential component of *motivation*, you can harness all the power and potential inside you and truly take control of your life.

THE NEW SCIENCE OF MOTIVATION

If human beings were simple, we would operate like most animals and be driven to perform only activities that aid us in two things: survival and reproduction. We would also eat only the amount of food we need to fuel our bodies, and we would conserve all our energy for defending our families and for hunting. Of course, we've evolved beyond such a simple, primitive existence and we visit drive-throughs (not because we're "conserving energy") to pick up food that provides more calories in one meal than we need in an entire day, and we consistently make choices that lead to a decline in our health without regard for the clear evidence of the dangerous repercussions. We make these choices because we can and because psychological motivators, of which

INSTANT INSPIRATION

"I remember what it felt like to be 195 pounds—having no energy, never wanting to get off the couch, and hating myself. That keeps me motivated to continue in the right direction. Every day I look in the mirror and see a stronger and more confident person."

—Tammy*vanyelmoon

many of us are unaware, drive us to do so. For decades now, behavioral scientists have undertaken the task of understanding how we make choices, and recently they've revealed surprising information about what drives us and the part motivation plays.

There are two types of motivation that I'll refer to throughout this book: fixed motivation and limitless motivation.

FIXED MOTIVATION: WHY IT WORKS ONLY IN THE SHORT TERM

Fixed motivation is what you will find in gimmicky fitness quick fixes; programs that operate within a narrow focus and consequently produce quickly expiring results. Diet or workout programs like this are often matched up with equally fixed goals, goals such as "lose 20 pounds before my wedding," "get ripped for summer," "impress my ex-girlfriend at my high school reunion." Sure, goals of that kind may initially motivate us, but they don't inspire or ignite true change, which means that once the event has passed, the muscles soften and the pounds pile back on.

Fixed motivation expires quickly because the initial goal setup is focused only on external rewards, things like grades, money, and appearance. Science proves that *purely rewards- or results-oriented goals like this don't create long-term commitment*. And it's not a matter of willpower, as you might think; it comes down to how we're wired.

I'm sure you recall the reward-and-punishment system used in school—good grades and gold stars for a job well done, a time-out or detention for a job not so well done. Whether you know it or not, those things were put into place to motivate you and help keep you on the right track. The same can be said about business organizations; we may grow up and leave school, but we essentially enter a similar system of encouragement in our places of employment, this time based on rewards of bonuses and raises and punishments of being passed over for a promotion or losing our job.

What the new science of motivation has shown is that, in truth, we really aren't that motivated by punishment, rewards, or surface-level results. Even money does not motivate us to strive; in fact, it actually stifles vital character elements such as creativity and persistence. Research has shown that children as young as elementary school age grow bored with superficial motivators; they are instead compelled to grow or learn when the rewards are things such as a supportive environment and acknowledgment.

One study tested a related theory by having two separate groups of college students play a puzzle game similar to Tetris. Researchers told one group that they would be paid for each puzzle they solved; the other was simply given the game to play. What happened was surprising—the paid individuals quit playing immediately once the experiment session ended, but those who weren't getting paid

continued to play the game beyond the timed experiment, simply for the sake of enjoyment. The monetary reward eclipsed the fun for the first group, and they lost their connection to the internal motivation to just play.

The same psychological devices are in effect when it comes to establishing health and fitness goals. Creating an initial fixed goal such as "I want bigger biceps" or "I want a flat belly" can, like a candy bar, give you a quick burst of motivation, but it fades quickly and results in a complete loss of momentum. To build ongoing momentum, you need to connect to limitless motivation, which comes from feelings of accomplishment, skill development, connection, and enjoyment.

LIMITLESS MOTIVATION: THE KEY TO LONG-TERM SUCCESS

The truth is, we really don't change that much as we get older when it comes to what drives us to excel at achieving our goals. As adults, we may think that the most motivating goals we can set are making more money, driving a specific type of car, or hitting a certain goal weight. But science shows that in truth we are actually motivated by the kind of intangible benefits—enjoyment, social connection, and a sense of accomplishment or growth—that inherently motivate us from birth. Focusing on fitting into a wedding dress or impressing someone at the beach with a ripped physique might get you to that goal in the short term, but it won't keep you there for the long haul. For that, you need to tap into a deeper system of limitless motivation.

When it comes to exercise and fitness, these more profound drivers trump the traditional results-based motivation every time. A study published in the *International Journal of Sports Psychology* compared "extrinsic," or external, motivators that were body-related—goals that were connected to improving fitness or appearance—to "intrinsic," or internal, motivators, which were related to competence, enjoyment, and social interaction. They determined that the second group of motivators proved significantly more effective in creating long-lasting commitments to fitness.

Another study found that even though many people begin diet or fitness programs to lose weight and look more attractive—because that's also what most programs promise—these

superficial types of goals tend to make them quit sooner and even minimize enjoyment; now, that's a lose-lose situation if I've ever seen one. We'll get more into developing your goals later, but these studies highlight the importance of strategically defining your goals—if you connect them to internal drivers such as self-confidence, skill development, and relationship building, you will increase your long-term motivation. I'll introduce you to the FLOW system for defining goals in Chapter 4, which includes creating goals based on both fixed *and* limited motivation, since one can give you the initial jump start and the other can keep it going long term. Here are a few examples of each:

FIXED MOTIVATION	LIMITLESS MOTIVATION
Get six-pack abs.	Get fit so I can play with my kids.
Fit into my skinny jeans.	Learn a new sport or skill.
Impress that girl at work.	Lose weight so I can have a baby.
Win a fitness contest.	Feel confident in my body.
Look great for a date.	Meet new people.

This may not sound revolutionary—that we like activities that are fun, prefer doing them with friends, and feel more confident doing something we've done before as opposed to trying something new. But until recently, these ideas have not been considered when creating approaches to fitness.

Research has shown that social support and connection can be important sources of limitless motivation, even helping people kick tough-to-quit habits such as smoking—in fact, people who quit smoking with even just one "buddy" are three times as likely to stick to their commitment. And if social influence can help someone kick a smoking habit, it can do wonders for curbing habits such as pushing the snooze button and skipping a workout! The key is to connect to this social influence within a solid fitness network, one that is grounded in the often neglected area of limitless motivation and includes powerful tools and information you can apply to your diet and workouts every day. I have seen people (inspirational individuals whom you will meet throughout the book) overcome struggles and issues of every sort, including alcoholism, eating disorders, disability, morbid obesity, insecurity, and time management conflicts by tapping into these foundational principles. You'll learn more about the actual steps of the Body by Design plan in the next chapter, but each part of the plan is based on this fundamental idea of tapping into your core of limitless motivation.

WHAT'S YOUR TRANSFORMATION TRIGGER?

Everyone I know who has found their own source of limitless motivation and broken their preexisting negative thought patterns has had what I call a "transformation trigger" that acts as the catalyst to change. Maybe it's a moment of public discomfort with your weight, such as not fitting into a ride at an amusement park. Maybe it's a more private embarrassment, such as realizing that you no longer fit into a pair of jeans. Or perhaps, like Captain Ahab, it was realizing you'd reached the ultimate breaking point with your body.

In my case, I had been training off and on for a while with mixed results, but I'd convinced myself that I was incapable of achieving my ultimate body, and this created weakness in my commitment. For some reason, I was fixated on my calves; it might seem silly, but I could never seem to get them as strong and developed as I wanted. And when I was presented with my true Achilles' heel—foods such as bacon, sausages, baked beans, fried bread with butter, and black pudding—the subconscious part of me that had already admitted to weakness made room for other doubts

INSTANT INSPIRATION

"Working out is a necessary part of my life, and it accentuates my artistic, competitive, athletic, and feminine nature. Most important, it makes me a better person as a whole."

—Juliet*JulietArtThou

and gave them plenty of space to grow larger. What initially seemed like a harmless bit of self-doubt opened the floodgates and completely obliterated my overall commitment to good health and fitness habits.

My transformation trigger was a friend saying to me, "I thought you lifted weights—why are your calves so skinny?" It was a small comment, but that was it for me. Something was finally triggered in my mind, and my thoughts went from "I will never have built calves" to "I will have built calves." By taking out just one word, I created a whole new pattern of thought. I'm proud to say that now my calves are my most developed body part.

I know that for some of you my story might seem to belittle the obstacles you're facing. You might be thinking *this guy just wanted bigger calves, and I need to lose a hundred pounds.* If you don't identify with my problem, there are dozens of other success stories in this book that represent the full spectrum of personal challenge—be sure to read all of them (you can also check out BodySpace on your own to scan through the hundreds of thousands of other stories there).

Let's shake off the comparisons for now and focus back on you—that's why I'm here, and that's why you're here. You are here reading these words right now and holding this book because you have arrived at your very own transformation trigger—this is it. Don't wait for the bad news from the doctor; don't wait for the embarrassing comment from someone at a party or in the grocery store aisle; don't wait until your kids are too old to want to spend time playing sports with you—start right now. In the next chapter, I'll show you how it's done.

In 2002 Errol Hannigan slipped on some grease on the floor and heard a pop in his knee. The injury was bad but not terrible, and he went in for arthroscopic surgery to have it repaired. "Simple day surgery is what the doctors called it," recalls Errol, who's known as Captain Ahab on his BodySpace profile. During surgery, the doctors overlooked a nasty infection that was building inside his knee. A month later, his doctors told him the infection was spreading. "It was moving up my leg so fast it would take my life if they didn't do anything."

Errol and his wife realized that there was no alternative but to let doctors amputate his leg. Two more surgeries later—bringing him to a total of seventeen operations—he was confronted by the most difficult obstacle he had ever known: phantom pain. "I had phantom pain 24/7, the worst pain I ever knew in my life," he says. "It went on for years. I just couldn't deal with it any longer."

On top of the high doses of morphine, Errol was self-medicating with large quantities of alcohol and food—gaining weight and spending most of his waking hours in a pain-fueled stupor. It was no way to live. "I got pretty low; *really* depressed," he says. "I couldn't take it any longer, so I lined a room in clear plastic and loaded my pistol and prepared to take my life. I went upstairs to say good-bye to my wife and ask for her permission to end my life. And she had just recently been diagnosed with lupus after years of testing. She said to me, 'No, I don't want you to take your life—I'm going to need you now.' So I went downstairs and unloaded my pistol and basically got ready for a life filled with nothing but pain and depression."

Errol's wife, Judi (read her story on the following pages), researched ways to counter the effects of lupus and decided that she was going to start exercising, which can help relieve symptoms of the painful autoimmune disorder. "Somehow she talked me into going to the gym with her—and I'll never know how she did that," recalls Errol. That trip to the gym changed his life forever. "Within five minutes of picking up a weight my phantom pain went away. Lifting weights brought him nearly three pain-free hours. "It honestly gave me a new lease on life."

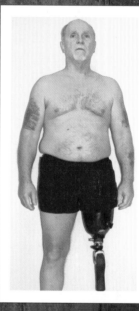

BEFORE

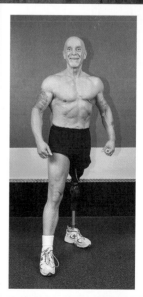

AFTER

Errol and his wife cleared their kitchen of ice cream, soda, and other junk foods, started eating six small meals a day supplemented by protein shakes, and stuck to a regular fitness regimen.

Despite having to deal with an amputated leg, Errol considers his life before fitness just like anyone else's: "My before pictures showed my muffin top; I was a donut-eating, self-medicating, wine-drinking, overindulging fat guy—I'm just like any other person out there."

He maintains that the path to fitness begins in the kitchen. But while cleaning out the cupboards was a top priority, so too was taking a social inventory. "I took a long, hard look at the people around me who called themselves my friends but who actually never supported what I was doing or acknowledged my progress," says Errol. "The ones who supported me I called 'Circle A' and made time in my day or week to connect with them. The ones who didn't support me I called 'Circle B,' and I all but eliminated those from my life and made a point of not spending time with them. I found that my life became a lot less stressful after doing this." He built up his "Circle A" group on BodySpace, where he has connected with and inspired thousands of others. "The support I have found online has been invaluable—my virtual friends help keep me accountable and motivate me to continue pushing for progress," notes Errol.

Now living a life free of depression and with minimized pain, Eroll has taken his passion for fitness and focused it on educating and motivating others. "I have a new outlook on life—every day is a joy," he says. "I want to lead the fight against obesity that is knocking down our countries. My wife and I have dedicated the rest of our lives to showing people that you can get fit and how easy it really is."

After years of dealing with a growing list of debilitating symptoms that included migraines, painful joints and muscles, and severe exhaustion, Judi Hannigan was finally diagnosed with lupus and firbromyalgia. "I had been told I had everything from the flu to it was all in my head, but the fact was that I could barely get out of bed," says Judi, whose BodySpace username is judimax. "I hated who I had become and was constantly worrying what the next symptom would be."

Judi had spent fifteen years working as an executive assistant, but her symptoms and eventual diagnosis made work impossible—"There was absolutely no way for me to work," she recalls. She fell into a routine that added weight gain to her list of frustrations. "I would wake up exhausted, have a piece of toast and then lie back down. Around eleven o'clock, I'd get up and watch some TV, have lunch, and go back to bed. Around four or five, I'd get up and figure out dinner, which was normally takeout, delivery, cereal, or cheese and crackers. Then I'd watch a bit of TV, eat junk food, and drink some wine, then go to bed." It was a depressing cycle with no end in sight.

Then, to make matters worse, something terrible and unexpected happen—Judi's husband, Errol (read his story on pages 13–14), after having his leg amputated, began experiencing devastating phantom pain, pain so unbearable that he came to her to ask for permission to end his own life. She pleaded with him and said, "You can't; I need you now." Judi hoped he would hold on to help her and that together they could somehow find a way to endure the pain. He stayed alive for her, but their future seemed bleak.

It was then that Judi's doctor suggested that she might get a bit of relief from her symptoms by working out. "Work out? You've got to be kidding!" she remembers responding to him. "I can barely get myself out of bed, and you want me to lift weights and go for a walk?" But she was desperate and started researching fitness plans. She decided to follow a program that recommended lifting weights three times a week and doing cardio three times a week. "I figured that I would at least be able to last that long," she says.

She pushed through the first four weeks for her husband, believing that was the only way she could get him to work out.

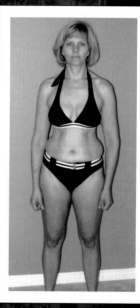

BEFORE

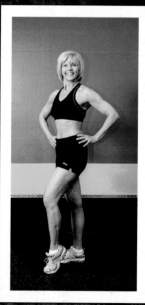

AFTER

> "The feeling of satisfaction, accomplishment, and the boost to my spirit during and after a workout session are worth every bit of the struggle."

"After that I started to realize that I wasn't quite so sore in the morning and I was getting a bit longer-lasting 'good' time," she recalls. "At about the sixth week I noticed a change in my body—I was losing weight and continuing to feel a bit better. Having tangible changes made me want to continuing going to the gym to find out how much I could improve." Instead of waiting for new symptoms to show up, she was taking charge and making positive results happen. Miraculously, Errol started experiencing relief from his phantom pain while working out; together they discovered fitness and unexpectedly transformed their lives.

Initially Judi relied solely on the support of her husband to keep her motivated, but then she discovered a way to add to her support team. "I got involved on BodySpace," she says. "The people there are real motivators to keep me setting new goals and working hard to achieve my current ones."

Judi also took a good look at the influences around her and made some changes; she started with the people who filled her phone book, then moved on to the things that filled her kitchen. "I eliminated 'friends' in my life who were not supportive and ensured that I only kept a network that I can expect support from," says Judi. "I also made sure there were no unhealthy foods or junk in the house." This policy remains in place today. "It helps when cravings hit as you only have good things in your cupboards or fridge."

While her symptoms persist and the process of just getting to the gym can present a daily struggle, Judi considers herself on the other side of a permanent lifestyle change. "The feeling of satisfaction, accomplishment, and the boost to my spirit during and after a workout session are worth every bit of the struggle—no matter how good or bad I feel going into the gym, I leave knowing that I gave my best and feel fantastic for it."

CHAPTER 2

The BUILDING BLOCKS of
the Body by Design Plan

There are a lot of things we can't control, including the weather, traffic, and other people's thoughts or actions. These can also be some of the most frustrating elements of life because they simply don't always do what we want. The good news is that there are parts of your own life that you *can* control. Connecting with your ability to practice control—and it is an ability—can be one of the most powerful drivers of change in your life.

I'm sure you've heard people talk about "self-control" or "self-regulation" before. It's the ability you think *other* people have that allows them to control how much they eat, drink, worry, exercise, watch TV, or—well, you get where I'm going with this—basically it allows them to control any behavior that beckons or balks at them. We also refer to this ability as willpower, which, contrary to what most people think, is not something you simply have or don't have (I'll address this in more detail in Chapter 3). One of my favorite books on self-change, *Self-Directed Behavior: Self-Modification for Personal Adjustment* by David Watson and Roland Tharp, talks about how we commonly think of willpower as almost a separate person: "Oh, you know, Will Power made me do it/not do it." The truth is, no one has or is lacking the willpower gene; it's actually something everyone can learn and practice, and it all starts with what you are thinking.

"Change your thoughts and you change your world," said Norman Vincent Peale, the author of *The Power of Positive Thinking.* You may think this statement seems overly simplistic, but you'd be surprised to discover how true it is. Science has revealed that our brains are incredibly impressionable, whether we are conscious of it or not. Researchers refer to a process called "priming," which is basically when your brain is set up to create an automated response. A study done in Amsterdam tested the idea of priming by having two groups look at different words before answering trivia questions. One group was prepped with thoughts of the word "professor" and the other "soccer hooligan." The "professor" group proved more successful in the trivia game. (While this brings in another layer about stereotypes and how they shape our responses, I want to focus on the power of thought demonstrated here.) Words and thought associations can assist the beginning of action, which I'm pretty sure is why you're here—you're ready to get fit and live a better life fueled by health, energy, and confidence. In this chapter, I'll discuss the basics of the Body by Design program that will give you the tools to do this.

THE FOUR PILLARS OF POWER

Starting in Part II, we will delve into the science that supports the core principles of the Body by

Design program: the Four Pillars of Power. You'll discover a little more about the motivational underpinnings of this program, and I'll share with you some more truly jaw-dropping client success stories, including stunning before-and-after photos. Each of the next four chapters will also include two transformational action steps. These are not to be missed, and I recommend that you make sure to follow the action steps as they're presented—they're strategically designed to build upon one another and help you maximize and fortify your commitment to your health. I will be here to coach you through each step as you move through the book.

When you discover and start to use the Four Pillars of Power, you will at last have the tools you need to turn desires into results. No matter if you're an adult or teenager, male or female, young or old, these foundations of motivation will ring true for you because they are linked to basic human psychology—we're all more alike than you think. I have seen inspiring transformations in an amputee, a 70-year old cowboy, a 20-year-old sorority girl, and a housewife with six kids, to name just a few—and they've all accomplished their fitness goals by applying the same foundational principles of motivation. Get ready to break through the limits of information and join the new fitness era fueled by motivational science.

The 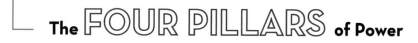 of Power

1. Burn and Build.

Bridges, that is. Research continues to pour in that proves the power of our social networks. Studies have shown that we are significantly more likely to be overweight or obese if our friends or family are, we have an increased risk of being a smoker if we hang out with smokers, and even that on a basic brain level, we are programmed to reflect just about any activity or behavior we see going on around us. That's why the first pillar is all about social inventory and how to identify clusters of influence in your life—and trust me, they are everywhere, including in your home, at your office, and even in the virtual social networks you belong to.

2. Live Out Loud.

Sure, you've been told before that goal setting is important; what you haven't been told is how to set the right kinds of goals—goals that set you up to succeed. You see, there are different degrees of power in goal-setting methods. Let me give you an example. Imagine you've decided you want to stop drinking so much beer (wine, cocktails, etc.) because, let's face it, it's not doing wonders for your gut. So the mental promise you make is "I'm going to drink only three nights a week." When the fourth and fifth nights roll around, that other voice in your head says, "Just one drink," and then that one turns into three or four, and on the next night you figure since you drank the night before, you might as well have a few tonight. Despite your original intention to cut back, you made a commitment with zero reinforcement and it failed. You'll probably agree that this is an extremely weak method of goal setting.

Your next step would be to write down your goal. So you write it on a piece of paper and stick it to the refrigerator; that way, every time you go to open it, you might think twice about that beer. Does this method work? We'll say it works better. The truth is, it works until something challenges you—a group of friends come over or you go to a party or just want to unwind after a long day at work doing what you know will make you feel better.

Then you discover how to create unstoppable goal adherence—you tell *everyone* about it. You share it with your boyfriend, girlfriend, or spouse, your parents and siblings, your friends and neighbors. From then on, every time you think about stepping off the path you've committed to, you have a whole reinforcement team to help remind you of your goal. If you make the same promise to thousands of people online—people who, even better, share your goal—well, then, there's truly no stopping you. This method of goal setting, what's known as transparent or public goal setting, is fortified and truly guarantees consistent success.

3. Get Radical.

Radical accountability picks up where goal setting leaves off; it ensures long-lasting suc-cess by providing the continuous feedback and guidance you need to keep you on track. I've experienced the benefits of radical accountability firsthand—when I was trying to get into top form and cut my body fat, I joined a BodyGroup (BodyGroups are user-created groups on BodySpace that unite people with specific shared goals). With about a thousand other people, I made a commitment to stick to my workouts and nutrition plan for twelve weeks. I've never felt more inspired and motivated than when I had this team of people who were depending on me as much as I was depending on them. We posted blogs, videos, and comments about obstacles and shared tips for staying on track. With this system of radical accountability in place, I not only met my goal but exceeded it—and continued making progress long after the twelve weeks were over.

Research shows that accountability motivates us for two reasons: first, once we've made a commitment known to other people, we want to avoid the sense of shame or embarrassment that comes from not being true to our word; second, we are driven by the desire for acknowledgment and encouragement—anyone who's ever run in a race or played a sport that included cheering fans knows how motivating positive feedback can be. Radical accountability also inspires healthy competition and encourages truly pushing yourself—if you see people in your support network set higher expectations for themselves, you are more likely to rethink where your limits lie.

4. Take It Home.

It's time to bring it all together. Life doesn't exist in a vacuum, and a true lifestyle change has to take into account factors outside your new motivational system of support. I'll show you *how* to change and not just *what* to change to make your new resolutions stick.

There you have a glimpse of the four proven foundational pillars of motivation that hundreds of thousands of BodySpace members have used to lose unwanted body fat and gain inches of muscle. Beyond that, these members have tapped into a system that inspires permanent change. These pillars are rooted in cutting-edge motivational science, and they each fuel one another toward a shared goal, acting as "force multipliers" that greatly increase your chances of success.

The BODY BY DESIGN Program

Of course, motivation alone isn't enough to get you looking and feeling great—you also need the diet and exercise to channel your newfound drive into tangible results. In Part III of the book, you will find a revolutionary twelve-week training and nutrition program designed to make your body over. Thousands of BodySpace members have already used these exercises and eating plans to create radical body transformations. You'll meet a couple of them in every chapter, and even more of them can be found online if you visit BodySpace.

WORKOUT AND NUTRITION PLANS: A SNAPSHOT

There's something in the technology field called "open source," which refers to software or other materials that are made available to the public for free in a way that it can be modified or improved by others. You've seen this type of system in action if you've ever visited Wikipedia to look up the biography of your favorite actor or the population of New York City. There is no one central source that supplies those facts—the information you find on the Wikipedia Web site has been created and edited by everyday people with a passion for information and knowledge. This empowering approach strips away the wall that once existed between "creators" and "users"—we are all creators in open-source technology.

Body by Design brings this open-source concept to life in the area of health and fitness for the first time. The program I'm going to present to you in this book isn't solely created by "Kris Gethin, Fitness Expert"—it has been compiled by a much greater living source: the hundreds of thousands of people on BodySpace who have undergone unbelievable transformations. The program in this book is a compilation of the best and most effective strategies used by these successful individuals, supercharged by me to ensure it delivers the ultimate in transformational power.

THE WORKOUT PLAN

There are three phases of the twelve-week Body by Design training program, each designed to keep the body guessing and prevent it from adapting to its environment. If the body adapts to its environment—the challenges of your workout—it doesn't evolve or transform.

1. The Fundamental Phase (Weeks 1–5)

During the first phase, I'm going to teach you the fundamentals of strength training. If you've never lifted weights before, you may be learning this information for the first time. And even if you're an experienced pro in the gym, you've probably been doing some things wrong, such as overtraining, and you could use a structured plan to get you back on track. This is your chance to focus on the fundamentals of strength training and set your body up for a profound transformation in the weeks to come.

The workouts in this first phase are designed to prepare the body for phase two using several mechanisms—it's not so much a rehearsal as the building of a solid foundation. We start out with isolation movements, which focus primarily on working a single muscle to prefatigue, and then add in a compound, or multimuscle movement that engages supporting muscles. By performing exercises in this order, we work the muscle to full capacity and separate development from one muscle to the next, which helps create a toned appearance.

The primary purpose of this five-week phase is to prepare the muscles, tendons, and ligaments for the heavier and more intense training of the second phase. During this first phase, you will perform three sets per exercise. You will gradually increase the number of sets

IN THE KNOW

ISOLATION MOVEMENT: Any exercise or movement that places stress on a single muscle or muscle group. Example: Bench Press.

COMPOUND MOVEMENT: Any exercise or movement that places stress on several muscles or muscle groups, thereby engaging an increased number of muscle fibers. Example: Squat.

FAILURE: The point in an exercise when you simply can't complete another rep while maintaining proper form (the key here is "proper form").

in the next phase, but by starting with just three, you can focus on establishing a comfort level with the form, breathing, and rhythm of strength training.

By beginning the program with all of these strategies in place, you will lower the likelihood of injury and maximize your body's ability to make progress and create stunning results. You will notice significant changes to your body during these first five weeks; while definition will happen a little further down the road, you will start to experience a toning of your muscles, especially if you're following the nutrition plan. Trust me, there's a lot going on with your body, no matter what kind of layers you have over your muscle; give it time, and you will experience an incredible difference.

2. The Momentum Phase (Weeks 6–9)

The second phase of training turns the tables on prefatiguing the muscle. This time, strength and muscle development is the priority, accomplished by completing a compound movement before the isolation. You will also be trying to reach failure in a lower rep range by using heavier weights. Remember, you've prepared your body for this in the first five weeks of the plan. The goal in the Momentum Phase is to add density to the muscle because the denser the muscle, the more calories are required and burned to maintain it—this is when your body starts to turn into a calorie-burning machine. Since more

assisting muscles are engaged, your body will also release more muscle-building hormones, especially in men.

You'll also see an increased training volume in phase two, which means you will be completing four to five sets. This will increase calorie burning, muscle density, and strength, and give a "rounder" appearance to the muscles.

Through consistency in carrying out the first phase, your metabolic rate will have risen enough to promote a much higher rate of fat loss, which works side by side with the muscle-building effect of phase two. The result: a dramatic change of appearance through muscle development and definition.

3. The DTP Phase (Weeks 10–12)

The last phase is an advanced cycle. By following the first two phases of the program, you will produce incredible results and you may very well have reached your goal by the end of the second phase. If you haven't, and you really want to push your physique to the next level, performing exercises using the Dramatic Transformation Principle (DTP) will undoubtedly take it up a notch. At this stage, I consider

INSTANT INSPIRATION

"You create your own reality and your own destiny—don't ever let anyone create it for you! It is possible as long as you believe it is. Developing my physique for me was like building a suit of armor to protect the frail sick little kid that I remember being."

—Chad*thenaturalone1ky

you to be at an advanced level and physically and mentally prepared for the three-week DTP Phase.

The exercises in phase three are very simple, but by introducing the DTP, you'll place a distinct stress on your muscles that will push them to produce previously unimaginable results—yes, you're going to want to show off a bit. The physical results develop so fast in this phase (assuming you're sticking to the cardio and nutrition elements) that I recommend you follow it for no more than three weeks. Due to the increased amount of energy required, if you continue beyond three weeks you run the risk of overtraining and wearing down your nervous and immune systems. By applying the DTP, which is a high-rep/low-rep method that will allow you to burn fat *and* build muscle, you will see results that you never thought possible.

In each of the phases you will find two supplemental sections designed to set you up for ultimate success: "Mind-set Motivation" and

"Physical Preparation." Be sure to read each of these before beginning the actual workouts— they'll ensure that you are prepared on all levels and help maximize your results.

CARDIO WITH A CAUSE

You will do cardio exercises throughout each of the three phases. While the duration will increase slightly as you go, the intensity, which is low, will remain the same. By keeping the intensity relatively low, you prevent your body from burning muscle for fuel, instead of fat—remember, you want to build muscle and keep it on because it will ensure that your body burns more calories at all times, even at rest.

I know a point of confusion for many people is whether or not to eat before doing cardio first thing in the morning. For this training program, I absolutely recommend eating prior to cardio, even though the advice in

WHY STRENGTH TRAINING?

When we get to the exercise chapter, I'll give you a full rundown of all the incredible benefits of picking up, and lifting, some weights (read "The Case for Weights" on page 88). But while I have your attention here, I want to point out that strength training is the perfect exercise for just about everyone.

Besides its long list of health benefits and ability to create dramatic physical changes, it is truly customizable for every person from any starting point. No matter how strong or weak you are, you can find a weight that works for you in the beginning and you can continually increase that weight to create new challenges and transform your body. If you want to increase strength, burn fat, build muscle, create definition, and tone, or look great in your jeans or on the beach, you can do it all with strength training.

many diets is to exercise on an empty stomach. What many of the experts who develop these programs fail to point out is that the body is extremely catabolic after an eight-hour fast and its metabolism is at its slowest point, which furthers fat loss and increases muscle wastage.

The sooner you eat upon rising, the faster your metabolism will speed up to digest breakfast; you will have effectively jump-started your body's fat-burning properties for the entire day. Food has a thermogenic effect, which raises the body's core temperature. Your first cardiovascular session of the day will be more efficient and productive if you eat beforehand because your body's fat-assimilating properties work much faster when they are under the influence of a thermogenic.

THE EATING PLAN

You simply can't hide from your diet; your body will reveal the truth—maybe not today or tomorrow, but I guarantee that the mistakes you make in your food choices will show up one of these days on your body, without fail. Sugars and highly processed foods will hold on to you for dear life, convert into fat, and conceal your potential physique from you and the outside world.

The good news is that there's a way to eat that will build your body's health from the inside out, eventually chipping away at that exterior layer and revealing the rocking body lying dormant inside you. To accomplish this, we'll stick pretty close to the principles of "clean eating," which include eating only whole, pure foods, avoiding highly processed or refined foods, and staying properly hydrated. This type of eating has roots in bodybuilding and physique athletes, but it now represents the core dietary foundation for most athletes and people who want to achieve top form. Not only is it the best for you when it comes to building muscle and burning fat, it is great for your entire body because it provides only top-of-the-line fuel for energy and the highest-quality materials for building new tissue.

The nutrition program in this book, which you'll read about in detail in Chapter 8, goes hand-in-hand with the training program and will provide your body with the foods it needs to simultaneously build muscle and burn fat. Straying from the eating program will only slow the progress of muscle building and fat loss; you may think that missing a meal or cheating here and there won't make much of a difference, but during the relatively short transformational time frame of twelve weeks, every meal counts.

INSTANT INSPIRATION

"I don't need to win; I need to move. I don't need to diet; I need to be healthy. I love how I feel after a hard workout, and I know that a clean diet is fuel for a great body—it's all about a healthy balance."

—Toni*tkatmommie

IN THE KNOW

CATABOLIC STATE: The destructive state in which your body breaks down tissue, including protein found in muscle, resulting in muscle loss and fat gain.

ANABOLIC STATE: The state required for body transformation; achieved by creating the perfect environment for muscle growth, which includes proper nutrition and adequate rest and recovery time.

THERMOGENIC: Heat-producing. Eating the right diet will increase your body's natural thermogenic processes by promoting the use of food as fuel over the storage of fat.

I'm going to recommend that you eat every two to three hours in order to keep your blood sugar level stable. This will help prevent cravings, increase your energy output, and keep your metabolism buzzing all day long. Plus, eating frequently will ensure that your muscles, which are depleted by your workouts, are given the nutrients that they need to rebuild and recover. You might think that eating six to seven meals per day will be a big inconvenience, but that's where meal replacement (MRP) shakes come in—these are packets of powder that you can easily store at home, in your car, in your desk drawer, or in a suitcase. Though they're not as good as whole foods, they are a safe haven and won't leave you stuck scarfing down a bag of chips or a candy bar when you're in a hurry. When you don't have time to prepare a meal, are stuck staring at a menu filled with junk food, or are at school or the office, these shakes can be a real lifesaver.

The eating plan is simple, but it's precisely what you need to transform your body. We'll concentrate on the two main macronutrients: protein and carbohydrates. You will consume fat as well, but only in naturally occurring forms. You will also cut out eating any starchy carbs in the last couple meals of the day. Since you won't have a chance to burn those carbohydrates off, you will remove them to minimize your chances of storing any unused calories as fat.

Since most of the foods I'm going to recommend are simple, pure foods, I'm going to offer you plenty of creative ways to add flavor and keep your meals interesting. I love to add hot sauces and ginger to most of my food, as I find they keep the body temperature increased, help spike metabolism, and slightly suppress appetite; and of course, they add great flavor. Check "Spice It Up" on page 122 for plenty of other ways to increase flavor without increasing flab.

The eating and training programs that I've previewed for you here will give you the map for success, but first you need to discover what's going to drive you forward: your motivation. So now we'll move to Part II, "The Four Pillars of Power," to lay the groundwork for your new, healthy life. I'm ready and motivated to get started on my own mission: to guide you through every step of this program. It's your turn to set the stage for your own head-turning success story. Get ready to transform your life!

"I'm a FAT GIRL Turned FITNESS NERD."

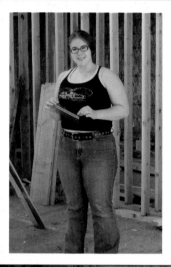

BEFORE

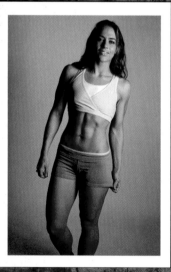

AFTER

"I weighed more than 235 pounds and wore size large men's shirts to cover up my body," says Tiffany Forni. "I had zero confidence and would constantly get taken advantage of because I felt like the only way I would be accepted was to do things for other people." Even though she had played ice hockey in high school, Tiffany's life at age 22 included little to no exercise, and her diet consisted of mostly fast food and pizza. "I was stuck in a bad cycle." She decided to go to a supplement store and get a weight loss pill. "I was a hundred pounds overweight and went into the store to ask if they had a pill that could make me lose weight without dieting or working out," she recalls with a laugh. "The guy at the counter said no and then told me about how bodybuilders eat."

She implemented the diet the guy at the store had quickly written out on a piece of paper for her. It was basic: eat every two to three hours; have protein with every meal; eat plenty of veggies; avoid fruit, dairy products, and refined sugars; and drink at least a gallon of water per day. "I tried it and lost 30 pounds in the first month."

Tiffany had never had aspirations of getting up on a stage in a bikini, but the progress she saw from her workouts and diet was inspiring. In the beginning, there were plenty of challenges. "Finding workout clothes that fit was my first challenge," she says. "Also, I have never been a morning person, so getting up to do cardio was not the easiest thing for me, but knowing what it did for me got me up every day!"

At first she kept her goals secret from family and friends, but she created a BodySpace to start tracking her progress. "I made my username 31233 rather than my name," she notes of her strategy to remain anonymous. "After a while I noticed that my progress was continuing, and I shared my profile with my friends and family."

She received encouragement from her boyfriend, family members, and fitness coaches, but she also found a support group of thousands of new friends online. "During my transformation the people I met on BodySpace became a great support group. All of the e-mails and phone calls from friends, family, and

BodySpace members kept me highly motivated to do the best I could," she says.

Losing more than 100 pounds and making a commitment to good health and fitness brought with it some realizations about who were her true friends. "The way some people treated me before my transformation was totally different from after—those are the people that I have since removed from my life," she says without regret. "The ones that treated me the same the whole time are now my best friends. It means a lot to me knowing that someone is not ashamed to be seen in public with me no matter what I look like."

It wasn't just her body that changed, though—her transformation has brought about new and inspiring goals. "I've learned that I want to help people. I've turned my life in a new direction," says Tiffany. "My goal now is to help as many people as I can change their lives through living a healthier lifestyle and losing weight. I want them to see that it's possible and know that their lives can be so much more fulfilling. I want to tell people that when life gets crazy and they don't feel like they have control over anything, the one thing that they do have is their own body and what they choose to do with it—recognizing that control can change your life."

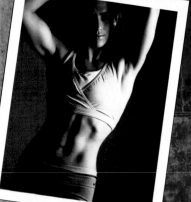

"My goal now is to help as many people as I can change their lives through living a healthier lifestyle and losing weight."

His HEART Almost STOPPED

Peter Czerwinski was 16 when a trifecta of serious health issues hit his family: his dad was hospitalized with bipolar disorder, his mom was diagnosed with multiple sclerosis, and Peter was told he might have lymph node cancer. He began to feel overwhelmed by the lack of control he had over the things around him. "I started to use food as a form of control to forget about negative things happening in my life. And then I took it too far."

Peter became anorexic and obsessed over nutritional facts. "I am not allowed to eat anything," he remembers saying to himself. He began to build up lies around his eating disorder. "I would wake up and figure out what I could eat for breakfast and then eat a fraction of that. I would then pack a lunch for school, which was usually a cucumber," he says of his daily routine. "I would get to school and keep to myself and not have any interest as to what was going on. Once I was home after school I would drink lots of tea because I was always cold as hell. Then I'd avoid eating dinner with my parents by constantly making up stories that I had already eaten, or I'd make plates dirty to make it took like I did eat." He eventually lost so much weight that he was down to 120 pounds, making his six-foot, two-inch frame look sickly and skeletal.

He was hospitalized with major heart complications; his heart had slowed to a point where it was barely keeping him alive.

After six weeks in the hospital, Peter arrived home knowing things had to change, and he quickly started working out and eating better. "I knew what I had to do to get better," he says, "However, on my own this would be a nearly impossible task. So I joined BodySpace and started visiting forums and began asking for help there and sharing my progress. I felt a lot more secure on there because I was a little embarrassed at first with what I was going through. In the real world, I didn't really talk about my goals."

Peter set up his BodySpace with the username "Dedicatedfor life"—he thought this would remind him every day that there was no giving up. He gained weight steadily and felt his confidence grow. "I was the shyest kid in the world before, but then I started gaining size, gaining knowledge, and simply becoming happy with who I was."

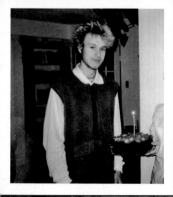

BEFORE

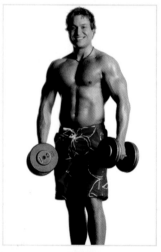

AFTER

One of the biggest keys to Peter's transformation was getting out of his own head and finding a way to tackle the negative and doubtful voices there—a step he recommends to anyone trying to overcome destructive patterns, which are often rooted in fear. "I think the biggest problem in this world is that people are scared of things that they are not familiar with," he says, "but the issue with that is they will never know if they actually are scared of them until they tackle that weakness."

Fears and weaknesses don't have to be tackled alone. "I don't think anyone is capable of achieving a healthy lifestyle and physique while hiding from the rest of the world. The more open you are, the easier it is to achieve your goals," says Peter. "A huge part of my success comes from using social networks and being open about my goals. Getting feedback from others who have been in the same boat is very motivating and comforting."

Fast-forward five years to a morning that would change Peter's life for the better. While at breakfast with friends he ordered "The Linebacker," a "two of everything" dish that no one is ever able to finish. When he finished the entire plate in what seemed like record time, his friends challenged him to keep eating . . . and eating. "I doubled the record in the hour time frame," says Peter of the four plates he quickly consumed. He had discovered a hidden talent for the most unlikeliest of things: eating.

Now a top competitive eater under the name Furious Pete, he has won thirty-six of his last thirty-seven competitions. "A big change from my life before is that not only do I eat, I eat better than almost anyone in the world."

When he's not eating competitively, Peter follows the basic tenet of eating when he's hungry, which, he says "just happens to be about six to eight times a day (but sometimes it's three or four). Most of my meals will consist of lean protein, healthy fats, and lots of veggies and fruit." By eating well most of the time, he maintains his commitment to fitness without letting too many rules overtake his life. "You don't have to diet your life away; just live the right lifestyle."

"You don't have to diet your life away; just live the right lifestyle."

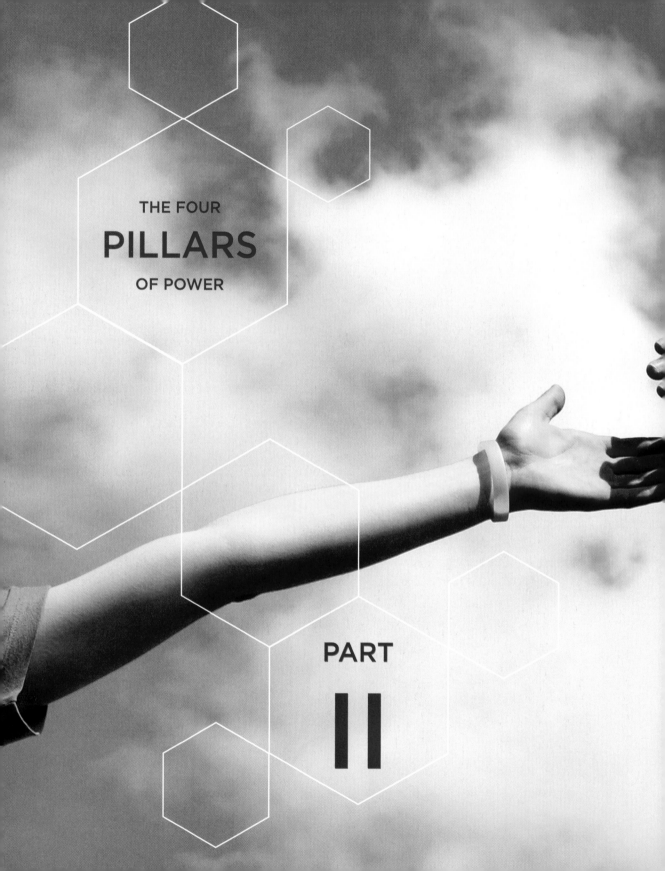

THE FOUR
PILLARS
OF POWER

PART

II

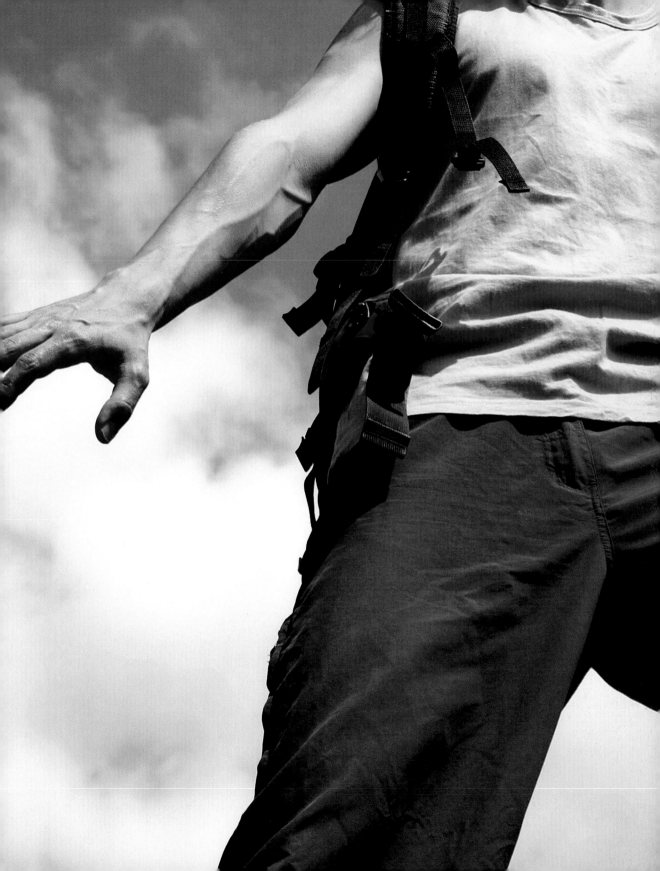

BURNING BRIDGES and BUILDING NEW ONES

I don't know about you, but I definitely remember getting into trouble for laughing when I wasn't supposed to as a kid—the quiet in places like the library and movie theaters is tough to take when you're young! It usually started because my sister or a friend started giggling, and no matter how hard I tried to resist, it took control of me, too. The same can be said for yawning—it truly feels impossible not to yawn when you see someone else do it.

For years, these kind of "contagious" behaviors were a mystery to behavioral scientists. What was most interesting was that they seemed to take hold in the subconscious; as one researcher put it, "It does not require conscious effort for an observer to imitate a yawning or laughing person." And that's not just science speaking; we know that's true because we've experienced it.

What they eventually discovered is that when we witness some behaviors we are unconsciously triggered to copy them. There's still some debate about how exactly this works in the brain, but it is thought that it may have roots in survival techniques. You've seen how when one bird within a flock breaks into flight, the rest follow suit. Though yawning, laughing, or coughing along with others won't save your life, they are adapted from innate behaviors intended to do so. What these shared experiences do is create a sense of belonging, which our tribal instincts always drive us toward.

Researchers have discovered that this type of mimicking also applies to behaviors that have deeper impact and significance, including even evoking particular emotions. The responses are activated by cells in our brains called "mirror neurons," which trigger us to imitate behaviors. We aren't the only ones who have this special ability; primates also have these cells, which compel them to copy movements such as reaching for food. In humans, mirror neurons are thought to be responsible for our ability to experience empathy, which means they help us have compassion, but they also make it possible for us to "catch" emotions just like a cold. Studies show that bad moods in particular spread from person to person like wildfire in the workplace, in couples, and among roommates.

What does all this have to do with your health? It means that even on a microlevel, the company you keep drives your actions and behaviors—without you even realizing it. The good news is this: an incredible potential exists because of this ability. We can learn, grow, and infinitely expand our lives by simply connecting with people who demonstrate positive and healthy behaviors. It's an almost superhero-like quality, and every single one of us has it.

THE MYTH OF WILLPOWER— EITHER YOU HAVE IT OR YOU DON'T

I would say we can all agree that some people just seem to have more self-control than others, whereas you might not agree with me if I told you that self-control or willpower is something you can actually learn from others. Let me tell you why this is true.

A famous study conducted decades ago on a group of four-year-olds tested what was thought to be an innate characteristic: self-control. A researcher at Stanford University named Walter Mischel created what's known as "The Marshmallow Experiment" to test how kids would respond when given the sweet treat. The researchers would put a child in a room and give him or her a marshmallow, with an important caveat: he or she could eat the one marshmallow immediately or could wait and be given an additional marshmallow to enjoy. As you can imagine, the temptation was nearly torturous for the kids, producing all sorts of squirming in chairs. Some of the kids gave in, of course, and others waited and received the extra treat, but that was only the beginning of the experiment.

Mischel caught up with the kids later in life to see if self-control played any significant factor in their lives. It turned out that those who had been able to delay gratification during the Marshmallow Experiment not only performed better on tests, they were more dependable, better able to deal with stress, and more skilled at problem solving—their willpower proved to have given them an advantage in life. What couldn't be determined from the study was whether or not this ability had been acquired through nature or nurture—in other words, could willpower be learned?

To test this, Mischel teamed up with another researcher by the name of Albert Bandura. They decided to try a similar delayed-gratification experiment, this time pairing the kids with a model demonstrating the skill of willpower. One group of children met with a real-life role model, and another group was given either written or verbal instructions supposedly left by this model on what option he or she would choose—wait it out or take what you get and go. Both groups of children, who had previously shown to be driven by the desire for instant gratification, displayed an "enduring increased willingness to wait"—they had learned self-control by simply seeing it demonstrated for them.

This brings me to your dinner table, your grocery store, the lunchroom at your office, the gym you visit (or don't visit), the teams or clubs to which you belong, the online social networks or Web sites you access—all the places that harbor role models who shape your decisions; like subliminal marketing, these forces guide your choices, for better or for worse and whether you realize it or not.

THE SPREAD OF POOR HEALTH HABITS

A groundbreaking research study was published in the summer of 2007 that revealed a potential underlying cause of the obesity epidemic. It was unprecedented because it did not simply point the finger at genetics or any one food or nutrient like so many other studies—"You're eating too much fat!" "You're consuming too many calories!" "You aren't exercising enough!" Instead, it considered an environmental factor we all share: a social network.

Researchers discovered, after evaluating

a large social network of more than 12,000 people over the course of thirty-two years, that obesity was quite contagious among friends. They determined that if someone considered a person a friend and that person was obese, his or her own chance of being overweight increased by 57 percent. If the friendship was deemed mutual, the percentage shot up to a 171 percent risk of obesity (the number is greater than 100 percent because some of the variables overlap).

The other incredible finding was that the percentage of risk did not change based on geographical distance, meaning it was not dependent on face-to-face interaction. It really doesn't matter if your overweight friends are in the same city or on another continent. It's possible, then, for influence to travel hundreds or thousands of miles without even having to jump on a plane—it's that powerful.

For some of us this will be a sobering—if not frightening—finding. Are we fated to be fat? Willed to be weaklings?

No.

Rather than looking at this phenomenon from a "glass-half-empty" point of view, I want you to flip your perspective. Sure, your social network can influence you negatively—but what if you think about it as going in the *other* direction?

THE POWER TO QUIT

About a year after the study on social networks and obesity came out, the same re-

searchers released another piece of powerful science. Published in *The New England Journal of Medicine* and called "The Collective Dynamics of Smoking in a Large Social Network," this second study considered the social group's power to pass along the healthy decision to quit smoking. If obesity spreads through clusters, would a positive health behavior also be passed along like a trend?

What the researchers determined created a collective sigh of relief in scientific circles—yes, it turns out that the act of quitting smoking spreads just like the act of gaining weight. When someone's friend, family member, co-worker, or significant other quits smoking, the chance of that person's also quitting significantly increases. While previous research had shown support networks or recovery groups effective at helping to keep people on track with a health commitment, it had not been studied in more casually formed social groups. The revelation suggested that the power of influence truly could be harnessed to create a sweeping overhaul of health habits.

There are many theories as to why behaviors are so often passed along through social networks. It could be that we are just quite impressionable—thinking back to the research about role models and delayed gratification, this seems a pretty valid theory. Or perhaps when we are exposed to something, we are more likely to accept it and no longer view it as strange or fearful. This is a pretty basic concept that relates to how trends of all kinds catch on: when something new shows up, whether it's a new style of clothing or a new kid on the block, we often approach with caution or doubt; as soon as we see our friends or, even better, a role model wearing something new or talking to the new kid, we want to jump right in. This idea brings us back to one of the core motivational drivers by which we are instinctually pushed into action: the desire to belong.

THE NEW MEANING OF CONNECTION

It is in our nature to want to belong; from an evolutionary standpoint, belonging meant we were part of a tribe, which in turn meant an increased chance of survival. Even though we have evolved beyond this sort of tribal dependency for survival, science shows that if we want to thrive as individuals and as a group, we should do it together. (Anyone who's tried to raise kids without parents or siblings nearby knows that it would be much easier with a "village" of support!) It seems only natural, then, that in the process of its own evolution, technology—the most dominant driver of

change today—has led to a reinvention of what it means to create connections.

I'll risk stating the obvious by saying that online social networks are everywhere. And not only are they everywhere, they are continually branching out and becoming more niche-specific. Because of this we can now connect with people worldwide who share our interests; we can find fitness enthusiasts, car collectors, fans of obscure music—you name it, there's a group out there that shares your passion, hobby, or interest. Like traditional social networks, our online versions have the same potential to be incredible forces for positive change.

Online social networks have been defined as "a fundamental part of the global online experience." Similar to other environments that shape experience, these networks and the members who populate them are influencers in waiting. Never before have we been presented with the opportunity to tap into such a deep well of motivation. According to research done at the University of Michigan, online social connections help spread behaviors, encouraging "transfers" of virtual gestures and tools.

This shouldn't be surprising if we think back to the research on the contagiousness of obesity—since geographic distance didn't make a difference in the level of influence, the friends must have been connecting via the phone and through letters and e-mail. (The study took place before online social networks

INSTANT INSPIRATION

"[The community at] BodySpace has been my *biggest* motivation. All of my friends on the site keep me going; these are ones who believe in me. I have never felt so good in my life. Working out is my daily drug!"

—Brittnie*LadyFirefighter

existed—if you can recall a time when MySpace, Facebook, and Twitter didn't exist.)

A lot of times people want to belong to social groups that are filled with members who are just like them. We find this appealing because chances are we are more likely to be accepted and not shunned by those similar to ourselves. While this comes from a place of self-preservation and protection, it can also be limiting because it shuts out chances for new and transformative experiences.

I want to make an important point about this because I think you need to hear it before we go through the action steps—*science proves that connecting with the right social network and system of support can provide the push you need into the action stage of change.* That means you stop thinking and you start *doing.* What you need to be aware of is the reality that a network may be filled with people with whom you don't immediately identify. They could be people who inspire you or whom you aspire to become. They could be like the people you've read about in this book, like Errol Hannigan and Tiffany Forni, who represent just a few of the thousands of similar stories at BodySpace.

BURN AND BUILD ACTION STEPS

In the Body by Design plan, we call this process of connecting with the right system of support "Burn and Build"—sometimes you have to burn a few bridges so you can make way for some stronger, more positive ones to be built. This is why Burn and Build is the first Pillar of Power I want you to discover—it's really the foundation from which all transformational change can happen.

I like to think of this process as starting with taking a mental "social inventory"—casting a wide net to see where the influences in your life come from. Then you can identify what bridges need to be burned and where you can reach out to build new ones. When I suggest "burning" bridges, I don't mean severing relationships entirely. I am referring instead to breaking down the chains of influence, which can happen simply by achieving awareness. What happens when you remodel your social network? You stop feeling stifled by your immediate social surroundings. I expect that for some of you, taking an honest look at the influences in your life will be a truly eye-opening experience—and what will be especially empowering is the realization that there are simple solutions to creating new connections.

This isn't just a matter of placing all the blame on others. It is important to hold yourself accountable for your actions (or inactions) and choices, but self-blame is not a constructive thought pattern. I want you to take a good, hard look around you. Stepping back to get the big picture will help you accurately determine what changes need to be made and where.

The best thing about reshaping your social network is that you open the door to limitless potential. On BodySpace I've seen this potential come to life in many of our success stories—people who've tapped into absolutely life-changing connections. In fact, one of the most powerful personal experiences I've had was gained by connecting with people there who have the same goals as I do.

Action Step 1:
Eliminate Negative Influences

I hope this chapter has opened your eyes to the fact that influences are truly everywhere in your life. Even though this step is focused on elimination, keep in mind that it is meant to be a realistic process based on your life; I know that some of the people who inspire poor health and fitness habits may be those closest to you. You can't run away from your wife or husband, parents, or best friend—and that's not what I'm suggesting has to happen (unless you happen to be looking for an excuse!). You can, however, make the choice to take control of your life. As I told you earlier with my own story, I was surrounded by people whom I had to get away from if I wanted to change my life—it was that simple. If you are in a similar situation, I hope you can use my story as inspiration. Realize you have the power to shape your own environment, and don't be afraid to lean a little more on the second action step to

help pull you out of your current surroundings.

When I use the word "eliminate," I want it to come from the power of awareness; you can rid yourself of negative influences simply by becoming more aware of their role in your life. Take your social inventory by stepping back to get a big picture: evaluate your friends, family, coworkers, social network friends, and so forth, and identify who drives you toward your goals and who distracts you from them. You can do this activity in your head, but personally I find that writing important thoughts and ideas down helps me connect with them better. Put the "drivers" in one column and the "detractors" in another; reserve the drivers for action step 2.

Once you have identified the key distractors in your life, it's time to eliminate the situations that allow for them to directly or indirectly guide your choices. If the choices are diet-related, be sure to become an active voice in decisions made around your home or office that involve food. (Check out Chapter 8 for guidance on transformational eating. You can also visit BodySpace to see what others are eating to lose weight and get into top shape.)

If the behaviors are fitness-related, I would guess that the problem is more about forces that motivate you to do nothing instead of doing something; it *is* tough to stop sitting on the couch when that's the predominant activity going on around you. Shake free of that unproductive and unhealthy pattern by checking in on your own expectations; if you are afraid to try taking your fitness level up a notch or you're overwhelmed by just the thought of exercise, you may be using others' inactivity to mask your own fear. Eliminate their influence and your own fear by creating microgoals—by starting small, you take control, and instead of focusing on the top of the mountain, you focus on each step you need to take to get there. For example, try committing yourself to exercising three days a week—no demands on how long or what type of exercise; just get off your butt! If your fitness level is more advanced, add specifics about time commitments and level of intensity. We'll get to more detailed and strategic goal-setting steps in Chapter 4.

Action Step 2:
Expand on Positive Influences

Now that you have mentally and/or physically prepared a clean slate, you're ready to expand on the positive influences in your life. First, I want you to reconsider the list you created and come back to the "drivers." These are relationships and connections you need to build upon, not eliminate. Maybe there are people on this list whom you admire and they push you without even knowing it, or maybe they've even invited you to come work out with them at the gym or play in a spontaneous game of basketball. You've never taken advantage of these positive influences—until now. Your first assignment for this step is to connect proactively with this person or people—send an e-mail,

make a phone call, post a comment—that's it, just reach out and make something happen for you instead of to you.

If you aren't fortunate enough to have those lingering drivers in your life, there are plenty out there just waiting to hear from you—they're hungry to show you the way. They are mostly people who have experienced such transformational change they have become evangelists for life and health improvement—you couldn't stop them from guiding the way if you wanted to. I'm talking about people like Tiffany Forni, who says on her BodySpace profile that her overall goal is to "help as many people as I possibly can to get themselves motivated enough to reach their goal." Or Michelle, username BuffMother, who signs off her profile page with "The key to your motivation is to encourage others." These are just some of the examples I've personally seen on our site, but there are so many phenomenally inspiring people out there, and with online social networks you have the power to connect with them.

The second part of this action step is to identify the social network that has the most members who inspire *you*. This can be a gym with trainers or members who have a level of fitness to which you aspire, a sports team, a weight-loss support group, an online social network, a walking or running club—you can even join a book or hunting club—the point of this exercise is to expand and grow your life and open it up to new potential. Ultimately, my goal for you is to realize this potential in optimum fitness; I can speak from experience when I say it will vastly improve your quality of life by giving you energy, strength, vitality, and surefire confidence (though I can't say whether or not a book club will give you all those things).

If you've never visited BodySpace, you are not aware of the numerous and incredible transformational stories we have there. You'll find thousands of members who are ready to take you in and guide you to a better life through fitness; one of the principal terms of our mission is "Motivation," and our members have really taken that on as their own mission, too—and I think you'll find plenty of it there. I invite you to check it out while you're trying on new social networks for size—it's completely free. Be sure to join the Body by Design group at www.bodybuilding.com/bodybydesign to connect with others who are following the plan featured in this book.

"My Life Was EATING, SLEEPING, and GETTING FAT."

Brad Spencer's life changed at a very specific moment—a moment so profound that he recalls every detail. "I was eating at a Chinese buffet, and I noticed a couple of tables away a young girl, perhaps four or five years old, watching me eat," he remembers. "The look on her face was not disgust or repulsion, as so many adults had; this look was sheer curiosity—I know that she had never seen anyone like me eat. Her parents tried to get her to stop staring at me, telling her it was not polite. She would look away for a few seconds, and then she would turn back to me, watching," he says. "Something in those few moments unnerved me—it was as if a key had tuned in my head. For the first time in years, I saw myself for who I was, and I understood that if I did not change, I would die from obesity."

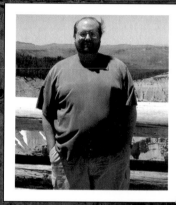

BEFORE

Brad went home that day and started reading everything he could about diet and exercise, but he knew he faced an uphill battle. "Mentally, I really believed I could not change," he says. "I had always admired and wanted to have a fit, muscular body, but I thought that I was cursed with bad genetics." Coming from an obese family with poor health habits, he lacked any understanding of what it meant to have a fit and healthful life. "We only understood one certain way to eat and live—there was never any exercise," he says, while acknowledging that the influence of friends and coworkers didn't help either: "I was surrounded by bad food and habits and friends who were more or less like me."

The moment in the restaurant pulled the transformational trigger for Brad; the next step was to take action by gaining control of his physical environment. "I got rid of all the unhealthy foods in the house, and I took the TV out of the bedroom," he says. "I used to spend the weekends just sitting around or staying in bed eating half the day while glued to the television—sometimes never seeing sunlight. My life was eating, sleeping, and getting fat."

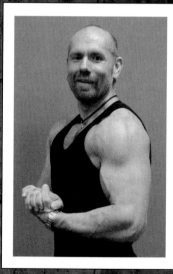

AFTER

He began by working out at home and, since he didn't have a strong support group around him with shared goals, making friends on BodySpace. "I found people there who were always helping me, answering questions, making suggestions, and giving me feedback." When he started working out at a gym, he made friends there as well and saw his relationships with his other friends who were obese or sedentary begin to change. "In time, negative friends—people who began saying I was changing too much—left, and friends who gave me unconditional support came into the picture," says Brad.

By losing 157 pounds Brad removed a serious threat to his life; since he suffered from nearly every obesity-related health issue, including high blood pressure, diabetes, and sleep apnea, the threat was beyond serious. The improvements to his health, though, marked only the beginning of the benefits of his transformation—he went back to school to study sports psychology and is now a personal trainer; he is enjoying the things that were a struggle for him before—going to amusement parks, hiking, biking, shopping in regular clothing stores—and he has a renewed sense of confidence: "There isn't a single aspect of my social life that hasn't improved for the better," he says.

Creating such significant change in his life took work, but Brad notes that one of the most important steps was a mental one. "The key to overcoming weaknesses or cravings is to admit far ahead of time that you have them—this seems obvious, but so many people do not admit them to themselves."

Another key: "Surround yourself with people who understand what you are trying to do and who can help you overcome," he advises.

When it comes to eating, he recommends two practical tips to everyone. "The two biggest changes to my diet were, first, eliminating any foods with added sugar—nature made things sweet enough," he says. "Second, I removed processed foods from my diet—with the rare exception, you will not find a box of food in my pantry—as much as possible it is fresh or fresh-frozen."

As for exercise, he emphasizes the importance of patience. "When a person is in the situation I was in, the key is to start slowly," he notes. "With cardio, I started out at five minutes per day, and I was slow with strength training as well—give your body a chance to adapt to all the changes."

> "The key to overcoming weaknesses or cravings is to admit far ahead of time that you have them."

Taking Charge to AVOID HER FAMILY'S HISTORY of HEART ATTACKS

With a family history of heart disease, diabetes, and obesity, Rochelle Ford knew she had at least one major incentive to improve her own health—she did not want to repeat history. "My mother has survived four heart attacks and my father one," says Ford. "Both parents also developed type 2 diabetes in their fifties from their lifestyle."

Ford says she had struggled with weight her entire adult life and that the struggle became even tougher after she had her daughter and couldn't get rid of the baby weight. "I was determined to make a change within myself," she says, "to take control of my life and reshape my body into what I wanted it to be."

According to Rochelle, one way to ensure you are connected to people who support your commitment to health is to find a social group filled with like-minded individuals. "I joined several online communities, but I chose BodySpace to share my transformation because I felt as if the members had a better understanding as to what I wanted to do and would not judge me but offer the support I needed while traveling this course," she says. "What I like about the site is that it does everything for you—it keeps track of your weight, measurements, body fat, and more—and the members on the site are truly great, too. I have formed incredible relationships and learned a lot from the people there."

After losing more than 100 pounds and transforming her body, Rochelle has a new sense of confidence and strength. "Growing up, I was introverted," she says. "I did a lot of listening and very little talking or sharing." When she made such a dramatic change to her body, people couldn't help but comment and ask questions. "With my weight loss, I've had so many people ask my opinion and advice about what they can do to get started on the same course," she notes, "which has forced me out of being that introverted child I once was so many years ago. I'm more confident now as a woman, mother, and supervisor."

Here, Rochelle shares some of her top tips for success:

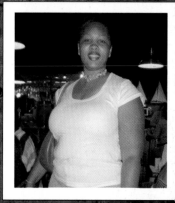

BEFORE

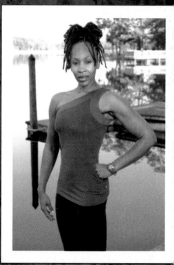

AFTER

➤ Drink plenty of water.
➤ Always eat breakfast.
➤ Feed your body at least every three to four hours.
➤ Eat lots of fresh vegetables throughout the day.
➤ Cut out carbs (rice, potato, and pastas) by 4 P.M. at the latest.
➤ Get creative with your meals and foods.
➤ Feed your body with a good daily multivitamin supplement.

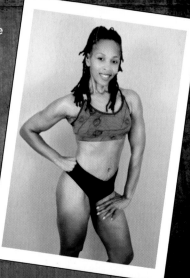

Rochelle's transformation has helped motivate others in her life. "My dad was taking several types of medications and was over 280 pounds at the beginning of the year," she says. "I began training him and showing him ways to change his unhealthy foods to healthier food choices. Just three and a half months later, my father is down by 37 pounds, walking more, exercising on a regular basis, mindful of the foods he eats, able to run steps, and has decreased the amount of medicine he was once taking. This goes to show that when we change our lives in a positive way, it can have a great effect on the lives of others."

The Power of OUT-LOUD GOALS

Without goals, you have no direction; without direction there is no incentive for action; and without action there is no progress. Simply put: your life minus goals equals settling for less than your potential. This is especially true with health and fitness, because even though every one of us is dealing with unique circumstances, genetic or otherwise, our bodies are designed to thrive. We all possess the potential to live a life filled with vitality. Your physical body is an incredible demonstration of cellular synergy, a complex framework of tissues that have come together to form organs and muscles, each of which performs incredible and essential functions. Your body *wants* to operate at its best, but it depends on you, the owner, to give it proper rest, fuel, and exercise. As I like to say, all bodies are created by their owners—treat yours well, and it will reward you for the rest of your life.

I want you to think about this now because this chapter is all about creating the most effective and powerful goals. I'll introduce you to simple strategies that make sense and, most important, work. When it comes down to it, though, if you haven't made the most fundamental commitment to being good to your body, you'll end up stacking promises atop a weak foundation—certainly not the right way to start things off. I have a quote by the motivational speaker Jim Rohn on my wall that helps remind me of this perpetual goal: "Take care of your body. It's the only place you have to live." Keep this thought in mind as we move forward, or go online and pick a favorite quote of your own.

The Body by Design goal-setting strategy will ensure that your motivation is fully ignited and will create a pattern of consistent behavior that unites you with your ideal self—you'll no longer feel a split between the person you are and the person you want to be. First, I'm going to take you through a quick exercise I call Prime Time—think of this as a few warm-up laps—and you'll discover the true secret of sticking to your goals: public proclamations.

PRIME TIME FOR SUCCESS

In Chapter 1, I mentioned the idea of "priming" and how participants in a study were prompted with words that created automated responses; I'm going to use this same concept to prep you for ultimate fitness success. Prime Time is another way of saying "mental preparation," which means you don't need anything for this process but your own mind—although I recommend writing down your thoughts if possible.

What are your self-defeating beliefs?

The first step of Prime Time involves recognizing your self-defeating statements, so I want you to think of all the words and phrases you most often use to describe yourself. These can be single words such as "fat" or "lazy" that float around you in little word bubbles or statements such as "I'm never going to get fit," "I hate my body," "Losing weight is for other people, not me," "I won't ever be able to create healthy habits."

Dig deep and be specific—what are the patterns or ruts of thinking that have you trapped? Even if you are already fit, this applies to you.

We all create an imaginary ceiling on our own potential—do you look at your butt or your arms and feel as though as fit as you get, you'll never look the way you want to? (Remember my calves? It might sound silly, but they were the bane of my existence, even though I was a pretty built guy at the time.) If you tell yourself that you have a "trouble spot," or if you believe that you're going to be too busy this week to make it to your workout—well, guess what, your body is going to believe it.

You've probably found people to inactively validate your doubts too (even though they don't know it)—it's pretty easy to find them (they are often part of the negative social network we talked about in Chapter 3), and letting them distract you from your goals is part of the destructive pattern in which so many of us unconsciously get stuck. Of course, there are people in our lives who *actively* validate our doubts or negative behaviors, but hopefully you learned how to eliminate the influence of those people in the previous chapter.

How do these beliefs play out in your life?

You've identified the negative thoughts and phrases that are holding you back, so for step two, I want you to consider the circumstances and scenarios that allow this pattern to perpetuate in your life. For example, since I had already convinced myself that I was incapable of achieving my ultimate body, this created weakness in my commitment—and weakness, like misery, loves company. Then, when I came

up against my ultimate weakness of fattening breakfast foods, that subconscious part of me that had already undercut my expectations was more than happy to encourage me to dig in. This kind of slip not only kept me from getting great calves, it completely sabotaged my overall promise to honor my body.

The problem in this underlying cycle of self-defeat is that it slowly eats away at your goals until you've surrendered them entirely; it's a slippery slope that all starts with a simple thought.

What is a more positive belief?

Step three of Prime Time is about creating the shift; changing the thoughts in your head from the ones that keep you stuck in a negative cycle to ones that perpetuate positive change. This can be as simple as turning the word "can't" into "can"—it's all about converting self-defeating statements into productive ones. If we look at some of the phrases I previously mentioned, we can see how easily they can be converted: "I won't ever be able to create healthy habits" becomes "I can create healthy habits"; "I'm never going to get fit" shifts to "I'm going to get fit"; "I hate my body" should be "I love my body." You may recall that for me, it was turning "I will never have built calves" into "I will have built calves."

If you don't think it's possible that such a simple step can have great power, I challenge you to try it and discover the outcome for yourself. Remember: if you don't truly commit to it, you are only cheating yourself, so genuinely practice a new thought pattern and witness the changes it brings about for you. Research shows that words and phrases plant themselves in our subconscious and drive action; I challenge you to take control and refuse to let your potential life rest on the back burner—let's fire it up!

How will you put that belief into practice *today*?

The final step will take us out of your head and into your physical environment. I want you to give primers a prominent presence in your daily life. Consider the words or phrases that inspire you and write them down on a sheet of paper. Researchers have shown that exposure to single words such as "strive" and "success" can subconsciously encourage perseverance and fuel motivation, so feel free to pick individual words or sayings.

Your primers can include sticky notes you leave for yourself in specific places that say GO WORK OUT or I AM AN ATHLETE or SKIP THE CHIPS— whatever statements you decide will support your new positive thought patterns. I've seen plenty of people put these kinds of notes on their refrigerator or on their computer at work—somewhere or something they pass by often. You can also tear out inspiring photos of beaches you want to visit while looking ripped in your trunks or toned in your bikini; or maybe of someone whose body you want to emulate.

Will these pictures and words motivate you forever? No. What they will do is prep your brain and, through repetition, drive your body to the point of action. To ensure that action is everlasting, you have to set goals strategically—which involves more than just you and your refrigerator. This is when you have to get loud.

THE POWER OF PUBLIC GOALS

"One of the simplest ways to commit yourself to a course of action is to go around telling all your friends that you are definitely going to do something," said Gerald Salancik, a prominent sociology researcher during the 1970s and '80s. Salancik based this statement on years of social behavior research, but if you really think about it, his scientific conclusion makes perfect everyday sense.

Let's consider my friend Ryan. Ryan's a driven, intense guy who appears to have no trouble at all maintaining commitments and promises he makes—to himself and to others. He sticks to his goals by being disciplined and focused, reading at least five books a week, eating well and exercising, being a good dad and husband, and pushing his business success to new heights. But Ryan one day hits a wall with a particular commitment—he's decided that he wants to cut red meat from his diet; he *loves* hamburgers and steak, but, for personal health and environmental reasons, he's decided he wants to eliminate it from his meals. However, he simply can't seem to stick to it. At business lunches, he orders hamburgers, and at home on the weekend he grills steaks for dinner. Each time he does this, he privately chastises himself for being weak and giving in. Ryan is stuck in limbo, or what's otherwise known as a state of goal conflict.

We face different types of goal conflict in our lives. They can show up in the workplace or at home—essentially anywhere there may be two or more goals that conflict with one another. These conflicts are tough to manage because they tend to involve outside forces, such as your boss's expectations or those of your significant other's. The goal conflict Ryan is experiencing, though, is one that can be overcome if he finds a way to unite his private thoughts with his public actions—if he can do this, he will break a destructive pattern that makes him feel defeated and frustrated.

The most powerful method to bind internal goals to external actions is to, as Salancik said, *tell everyone about your goals*: in other words, to make your private commitments public. Studies have shown that turning a private goal into a public one can propel it from a passive to an active state; like the flip of a switch, sharing your goals with others shines a light on your commitments and ensures that you stick to them. It may seem as though a simple concept couldn't possibly have such a significant impact, but research has repeatedly proven that telling others about your plans can make all the difference.

When social scientists tested this theory on a group of women trying to lose weight in India, they determined that those in the group who made their commitment public not only lost significantly more weight, they were also able to make their commitment long term. For the most successful women in the group, sharing their goal to lose weight with others provided the motivation they needed.

Ryan found this to be true for him, too. He told his wife and coworkers about his goal and gradually worked it into most conversations to make sure his commitment was widely known. Before he knew it, he had a whole team of people helping to keep him on track.

Now, the interesting thing here is that this type of impact is created without any action needed from others—the people who heard the women's goals in the study or the business partners who discovered Ryan was committed to cutting out red meat were passive enforcers, not active ones. All the work was done by those who were sharing their goals—and sharing was the only work required.

What happens when you make a visible commitment is that you put your reputation on the line. If you share a goal with someone and then act inconsistently with fulfilling it, you are seen as lacking integrity and trustworthiness. If Ryan started eating a hamburger at lunch after just having shared his goal publicly, he would have been perceived as weak and revealed cracks in

> Like the flip of a switch, sharing your goals with others shines a light on your commitments and ensures that you stick to them.

his character. This isn't just an example of caring about what others think of us, it's actually a survival adaptation. We inherently strive for a sense of belongingness because we have been brought up in families, tribes, and communities; sticking close to these groups has always meant an increased likelihood of survival.

One famous recent example can be seen in the story of Julie and Julia. In her best-selling book, and later in the feature film of the same name, Julie Powell was driven to complete her goal of cooking her way through Julia Child's *Mastering the Art of French Cooking* within a year because that was the goal she had set for herself on her blog—and she knew people were watching her and rooting for her.

We've also seen this appear in the form of the "public apology"—every publicist's nightmare is also a perfect example of the power of public proclamations. Once Tiger Woods and Jesse James issued public apologies and promises to change, they, whether they liked it or not, had enlisted a country of onlookers who were eager to see them remain true to their word—their credibility was officially, and very publicly, put on the line.

I'm going to have you apply this same strategy to prevent cheating—on your diet—and help you create a solid commitment to your fitness goals. Long-term motivation for goal pursuit also comes from connecting your goals to internal drivers such as confidence, skill development, and relation-ship building instead of limiting them to just surface-level accomplishments such as getting ripped abs or losing 20 pounds.

I hope you've prepped yourself for success by dedicating a bit of time to Prime Time. With the following action steps, I'm going to teach you how to define your goals strategically and then give you the tools to declare them. Think of this as planning a dream vacation to visit your new life (although I think you're going to want to stay there permanently, so pack accordingly!). First you're going to establish the destination and all its attributes; then you're going to take the first step toward getting there by telling all your friends where you're headed.

PUBLIC GOALS ACTION STEPS

Action Step 1: Define Your Goals

I know I've talked a lot about the mental roots of change and how motivation and strategic goal setting are essential to your success, but I want to bring the idea back to the surface for

INSTANT INSPIRATION

"Internally, I value my health because I know that it grants me independence. Living a healthy lifestyle helps me appreciate the aging process because I can continue living an active life."

—Pat*patbanya

a moment because, let's face it, some things can be said without science: you want to look good. I get it, and I want to make sure you know that as your guide and coach through this program, I have not overlooked this important desired outcome.

Let me make something clear: the Body by Design nutrition and training elements will ensure that you achieve your physical goal—you're going to look incredible—but that's just the beginning. My personal goal for you and your experience with this program is that you will undergo nothing less than a true transformation; that you'll emerge from this program with a dedication to a better life, to your *ideal life*—one that you exist in with such happiness, fulfillment, confidence, and satisfaction that you will never look back. I'm talking about way more than just great glutes—but those will look pretty good, too.

When it comes to defining your goals, the most important starting point is to establish that *you* are responsible for you goals—you are making the choice and the commitment to fitness; this transformation is for you, and it will be created by you. If you don't truly connect to this commitment and take ownership of it, it won't last.

I want to return quickly to the idea of fixed motivation versus limitless motivation before we establish your specific goals. You'll recall that fixed motivation focuses only on surface-level goals—such as, for example, "Add two inches to my biceps." Limitless motivation comes instead from goals that are connected to areas of deeper fulfillment, such as enjoyment, skill improvement, and personal accomplishment. The difference between the two is that fixed motivation stems from extrinsic (outer) goals and limitless motivation originates from intrinsic (inner) goals; I like to think of intrinsic goals as those that answer the question "*Why* do I want to get fit?" Research has shown that outer goals aren't useless—in fact, they can provide the initial kick start—but they won't keep the fire burning for long.

To generate true and absolute goal commitment, I'm going to have you set your goals using **FLOW**—they should include a **F**ixed goal, a **L**imitless goal, **O**pportunities you will gain by pursuing or achieving your goal, and **W**eaknesses that may sneak in and try to sabotage your success. I've designed this system to ensure that your momentum will be swept up in a current of lasting commitment—with a solid goal foundation, there's no looking back.

INSTANT INSPIRATION

"Setting minigoals keeps me motivated. Not only do I enjoy reaping the benefits of whatever goal I have just accomplished, but the act of reaching that goal makes me feel amazing. When I set out to do something and achieve it through hard work, it is a personal satisfaction unlike any other."

—Sarah*oceanblue149

Let me show you how to use a FLOW Chart by setting my own goals using the system. Here's how mine would look:

Fill out your own FLOW chart on pg. 192.

You'll notice that the fixed goal connects to an appearance-related outcome; the limitless goal to things that will inspire me from within; opportunities relates to the new doors that will open to me as I continue my commitment to health; and weaknesses lays out the potential roadblocks that may pop on my path to good health. Set your own goals by writing them down in a journal or using the blank FLOW Chart on page 192. Fill it out and put it up on your bulletin board or refrigerator—or create your very own BodySpace profile online and add your goals there. I encourage you to add them online or share them with your friends and family because that will truly reinforce your commitments. Speaking of sharing your goals with others, let's move on to step two: Declare Your Goals.

Action Step 2: Declare Your Goals

Declaring your goals is all about reinforcement; it's an invaluable step with immense power, and the crazy thing is, it requires very little effort from you—you simply have to pass out your cards.

Passing out your cards is another way of saying sharing your goals with others. The phrase comes from a story I read about in a fantastic book called *Influence: The Psychology of Persuasion* by Robert B. Cialdini (though technically a business book, it provides some incredible insights into what makes people tick).

Dr. Cialdini shared a story about a woman he met who was continually trying to quit smoking. After reading yet another study about how smoking causes cancer, the woman, whom we'll call Suzy, said she was once again thinking about trying to quit. She decided that this time that she would indirectly recruit support from people in her life. To do this, Suzy took out several blank business cards and wrote on them a simple message: "I promise you that I will never smoke another cigarette."

She mailed the cards to friends and family, passed them out to others, and let the invisible forces of her character go to work—she knew that she simply couldn't go back on her promise now that others were aware of it. "There must have been a thousand times when I thought I had to have a smoke," she said. "But whenever that happened, I'd just picture how all the people on my list would think less of me if I couldn't stick to my guns. And that's all it took. I've never taken another puff."

So how or why was it that these cards were able to help Suzy quit one of the most addictive habits around, a habit that millions try to kick with patches and prescriptions, only to repeatedly fail? She tapped into the power of public commitment, as Ryan did when he was trying to quit eating red meat and like

countless of others (including thousands of BodySpace members) have done to help keep them on track.

Making a goal public doesn't involve airing your dirty laundry or even revealing anything too specific about your goals. In fact, one research study that tested the effectiveness of a public commitment to weight loss determined that the only information needed was a person's name and how much weight he or she wanted to lose; the person didn't have to post a picture or reveal anything else to tap into the motivational source. Of course, the more you are willing to put out there, the more you will get back, but what's encouraging about this study is that it doesn't take much to start—yes, this is me, stamping out your excuses one by one.

The power of public goals has been studied in many different settings, including movements that have created social change. Researchers have found that public commitments to do things such as conserve energy, stop littering, or start wearing seat belts have been critical catalysts in creating the spread of behavior change—kind of like the contagious yawn, on a much larger scale and with a much more significant impact.

In the beginning of this book, I mentioned the Body by Design program and how it's rooted in a genuine fitness movement—BodySpace, where there is a virtual universe filled with individuals who have transformed their lives and are waiting for you to join them. But the truth is, it could be at BodySpace where you track down the people who will help you change your life, or those people could be your family, your friends, your neighbors, your friends on Facebook, or people at your church or your kid's school—regardless of the group, the initial step of sharing your commitment to fitness has to come from you.

Before you start sharing your goals, though, I want to give you three final things to keep in mind based on social behavior research. First, sharing your goals with people you can relate to will maximize the strength of your commitment. Second, if you have confidence in the system of support and the tools you've received, you are more likely to be successful (I've got you covered with the "tools"—in Part III, you'll find everything you need for training and nutrition). Third, remember that you don't have to limit yourself to the people in your immediate surroundings—studies show that even distant connections can have a significant impact on your habits.

So now's the time for you to break out of your private space and take it public; it's a simple step toward a big change that you can take right now.

LEADING BY EXAMPLE

Antonio Wright always had issues with his weight; even as a small child, he remembers being referred to as "stocky" and "big-boned." But it wasn't until he was a few years away from turning thirty that it began to bother him. "I was looking in the mirror at myself, and I was disgusted at what I was seeing," says Wright, otherwise known as AntonioWright on BodySpace. "I was ashamed that I had let myself get to nearly 300 pounds."

Although those feelings about his weight were tough to handle, he experienced his true transformation trigger at a very specific moment—when a girl rejected him by saying he was "too fat" to be seen with her in public. "That was all the motivation I needed—if I was going to be rejected for anything, it wasn't going to be because of my weight!"

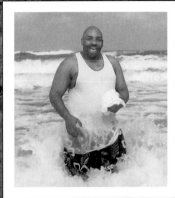

BEFORE

He had tried getting fit before but had focused on cardio and ended up looking what he calls "skinny fat"—thinner, but with no muscle tone or shape. Wright knew that to make a real change to his body, he would have to hit the gym. "I know some people struggle with going to the gym at first because they're intimidated," he says, "but ninety-nine percent of the people want to get a job done and get out of there—they don't care what anyone else is doing."

When it came to eating, Wright made some immediate changes: he stopped adding sugar to anything, eliminated all fast foods, and cut out iced coffee drinks filled with sugar and breakfast pastries, which included putting an end to his twice-daily visits to the local Dunkin' Donuts, where, he says, "I visited so frequently, they knew me by my first name!"

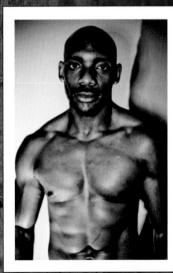

AFTER

In addition to making significant changes to his diet and exercise habits, Wright made sure his goals weren't a secret. "I told everyone who would listen!" he says. "The more people who know, the more you're held accountable. You're not on some secret mission here—you're trying to change your life, and you're going to need all the support you can get."

To help him stay on track, Wright tapped into the deep well of resources and support at BodySpace. "The BodySpace forums and connections I made provided all the support I could ever need! You need a support group when you feel down; you need to hold yourself accountable when you slip up; and you need to be transparent with all your actions, because you can fool yourself, but you can't fool everyone else."

When he first started out on his transformation, Wright made sure to give himself a cheat day, but more for psychological reasons. "At first I needed to know that that day was going to be there," he says, "but then I actually stopped craving bad foods. When you start eating nutrient-dense foods, unhealthy foods just don't taste as good. And the funny thing is, you might think you're going to be hungrier when you're eating well, but I actually have to remind myself now that it's time to eat."

Wright cooks nearly all of his meals at home to help make sure that he's in control of the ingredients that are fueling his body. "I've got a little cooler bag with a shoulder strap that I fill with my meals for the day and bring with me to work," he says. When he and his girlfriend are going to go out to eat, they plan ahead to avoid impulsive ordering based on hunger. "We look at the menu online if we can and decide what we're ordering ahead of time."

After losing more than 100 pounds, Wright considers himself firmly planted in his new lifestyle but maintains that the mental focus has to remain a permanent fixture. "My body is definitely working against me—it wants to be fat," he says, "but luckily the mind is the most powerful muscle in the body. Most of our weaknesses are mental, and they can be overcome with time. I have cravings just like everyone else; however, I look at the big picture."

He also finds constant motivation from knowing he's inspired others. "I receive so many e-mails from people who I have inspired," says Wright. "While they all are important, the most important has been seeing my mother go through her own transformation. And now my father is getting into working out—leading by example is the best method of teaching, in my opinion."

"I AM NOT HIDING Out Anymore
Being a 'Closet Eater' and Feeling Depressed."

When a coworker was let go, Monica Gregerson had to take on the extra workload left behind. What she also ended up taking on was an extra 55 pounds. "I was so worn out from work stress that I gradually stopped caring about my own health," she says. "Working out and my healthy diet were replaced with fast food and occupying space on the couch after work."

Even though she knew her habits had changed, it wasn't until one day when she went to put on her jeans that she realized the impact. "I had noticed that my clothes were getting tighter and tighter along the way, but it wasn't until one day I went to put on a pair of jeans and they no longer went over my thighs—I had to go to the store to buy larger jeans," she says. "I tried size ten, but they didn't fit. Neither did size twelve, and size fourteen wasn't looking too promising either. When I still had issues with size-sixteen jeans, it hit me hard as to how much weight I had really gained. I didn't buy the jeans that day; I went home instead and vowed to make serious changes."

Monica started eating healthful meals every two to three hours and working out regularly. The changes were quick to reveal results; she lost 20 pounds in the first month.

"Then I had an incident at work where I fell down twelve or fifteen stairs and was not able to train at the gym for nearly a month," she says. "After recovering from that fall I started training again but quickly hit plateaus, and it became frustrating to me. That's when the mental roadblocks showed up. When you stop seeing changes, you can get into a frame of mind of 'If I eat one more cheeseburger it's not going to matter.'" She says this is the precise moment when stepping back to gain perspective is critical. "It's now time to remind yourself that you did not gain this weight overnight and it certainly isn't going to come off overnight."

Even though she had support from her friends and family, Monica was excited to discover an even stronger source of support in her connections on BodySpace, where she's known as mongre78. "I have to say that my friends there were my biggest

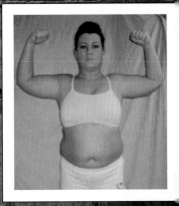

BEFORE

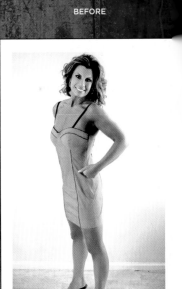

AFTER

supporters," she says. "I've made friends there from all around the world, people of all different shapes and sizes with many different goals."

Making her transformation happen also included taking inventory of her own weaknesses and developing strategies to overcome them. "I realized that my weakness is sweets—junk food like pop or candy—all the things my body did not need," she says. "I can't have just one Oreo, I have to eat the entire package! So I developed a motto, which is 'All or nothing.' And I choose nothing because I feel so much better without those things. And once I had the junk foods cleaned out of my system and I had replaced them with healthier options, I felt so much better," she says. "After going without those things, you don't even have a desire for them anymore."

She now eats five meals a day that are spaced every three hours. "I think this is one of the most important aspects of your transformation," she says. "By continually fueling your body with healthy food, you will stay energized and won't get hunger temptations. Also, take a great multivitamin and drink lots of water." To help eliminate any excuses, Monica always makes sure to prepare her meals in advance.

After losing 57 pounds and transforming her body, Monica has discovered a new life filled with nonstop activities. "Since my transformation I am out and about much more," she says. "I love being outside doing physical activities, such as running and playing team sports." Her active life is also one filled with a renewed sense of confidence. "I enjoy time with my friends much more because I am not struggling with low self-esteem," she notes. "I am not hiding out at home anymore being a 'closet eater' and feeling depressed. I have so much energy and I do so much every day—I am incredibly thankful that I am healthy and able to enjoy my life!"

CHAPTER 5

Get RADICAL

Take a look at these two statements and think about the difference between them: "I write." "I'm a writer." What stands out to you? The first is just a statement of an action, and it could be applied to any hobby or activity you engage in. The second, however, has a bit more significance—it establishes an identity and suggests an ongoing commitment to the activity as a way of life.

Now let's consider this as it relates to health and fitness— how many people can say they've dieted and worked out at one time or another in their lives? I would guess just about everyone. Considering that there's a term for bouncing into and out of food health—yo-yo dieting, which should also include yo-yo exercising—I'd say it's pretty common. The problem here is that a commitment to health and fitness should not be treated as casually as trying to decide on your favorite brand of jeans. Fitness should not be your fair-weather friend, it should be and *can* be a lifelong one.

Inconsistent commitments to health and fitness leave a greater physical and mental toll than you may be aware of. Regaining weight after losing it puts an increased strain on your body and only worsens conditions such as high blood pressure and high cholesterol. On top of the physical impact, the psychological stress is equally burdensome—weight fluctuations can cause feelings of guilt, shame, embarrassment, and frustration and inevitably contribute to a decreased sense of overall well-being.

So what's missing? Why is it so many people spend time drifting into and out of diet and fitness programs without ever creating a lasting connection to health? They're missing the vital element of accountability.

RADICAL ACCOUNTABILITY: THE SECRET TO MAKING IT STICK

Radical Accountability picks up where goal setting leaves off by giving you the continuous feedback and guidance you need to stay on track. When you establish your goals within a framework of accountability, you further reinforce your commitment to improving your health and quality of life. And I'm not just talking about avoiding disease here; I'm talking about living the best life possible. I'm talking about living a life fueled by strength and energy, one that doesn't just allow you to scrape by and barely pass a health test but enables you to say, "This is the best I've ever felt in my life!"

To be held accountable is to be kept on track; measures of accountability act like glue by keeping you stuck to the steps that will lead you to goal fulfillment. The sense that someone or some kind of system is always there is motivating from both avoidance and reward perspectives—once accountability structures are in place, we want to avoid the embarrassment, disappointment, or shame that comes with a lapse; on the flip side, we are driven by the potential rewards of acknowledgment and encouragement if we follow through on our commitments.

INSTANT INSPIRATION

"I am motivated by those who say that I am an inspiration to them and those who say reading about what I have done motivates them to push themselves harder. How could I not be motivated by those words?"

—Errol*Captain Ahab

INSTANT INSPIRATION

"Everyone on BodySpace motivates me. When I look on [the site] and see someone more defined than me, I love it; it makes me push harder and try harder. When I get asked advice, I love to give it and it makes me keep doing the things I do!"

—Elijah*SuperMaine

Researchers have tested the merits of accountability in different environments, but they've paid particular attention to the area of addiction recovery. While addiction is a very serious problem with destructive power, the behavior patterns that enslave addicts are the same ones that can create personal ruts related to general health habits. The repercussions may be less severe, but ultimately living a life without commitments to health and fitness can have serious consequences—poor diet and lack of exercise have consistently been linked to increased risk for disease and even premature death. Or, as someone in a white coat put it, "[The] pattern of exercise relapse is similar to the negatively accelerated relapse curve often seen in addictions."

The good news is that strategies used to treat patterns seen in addiction have proven effective in interventions related to health habits. The goal in either case is to reach the stage of maintenance, or the point where you don't intend to change back to your old ways. This is the point when the high obtained from working out is what you look forward to instead of the lull of the couch—when, as successful main-tainers in one study said, foods such as candy and doughnuts are "no longer appealing because [they're] too sweet or fatty." Does this seem unfathomable? Read on.

In many cases, continuous feedback from the right support system has proven to be the key factor in creating maintenance. One study looked at a group of people with diabetes who faced the difficult process of changing their health habits, including regularly monitoring their blood glucose. Researchers paired individuals who were struggling with adopting new habits with those already in the maintenance phase—people who had successfully formed new habits and no longer found the necessary health practices to be difficult; rather, they considered them to be automatic, like brushing teeth or driving a car.

For eight weeks, they followed a "buddy system"—the coach, or already successful individual, would check in with the newcomer and answer any questions, address struggles, and offer words of encouragement and a sense of companionship. The coach was also available to offer help whenever it was needed. This system of support and accountability proved incredibly effective, with all the newcomers saying that their "consciousness had been raised" and that they planned to continue with all the new health habits in place.

This system of accountability worked for a number of reasons: the continuous feedback, the sense of bonding created by connecting with people who have similar goals and struggles, and the optimism and confidence that come from witnessing success—*if they can do it, I can do it!*

Now I want to point out an interesting side note about this study because it connects to the different types of motivation that we've talked about in this book. All the participants in this study were being paid to participate, but by the end they had forgotten and "acted very surprised when they received their payment at the final focus group." The intrinsic drivers are ignited when we're inspired by things such as connection and learning. They were so powerfully revved in this experiment that they made people forget entirely about the "external" motivation of cold, hard cash.

Researchers have shown that this framework of support is effective in helping people quit smoking, stick to commitments to eat more fruits and vegetables, and manage their weight long term. I've seen this power demonstrated again and again on BodySpace—especially in the BodyGroups, which, you may recall, are user-created groups that bring people with similar goals together. I have taken advantage of the solid peer feedback offered in these groups many times—they never fail to keep me pumped up and on track.

HARNESSING THE POWER

In light of the current obesity epidemic, health institutions and organizations are scrambling to find ways to influence people to change, but the ranks of those crippled by poor health continue to grow. I say it's time to take the problem into our own hands by connecting as a global community; it's time to start relying on one another and using the power of our social connections to spread good health habits and happiness.

A government-sponsored report on obesity acknowledged the high cost of "lifestyle interventions" aimed at helping people create new health habits. It referred to the "growing crisis" of obesity and the great need for public health and policy solutions. Basically it said that we've got a huge, expensive problem on our hands with no real solutions in sight. But let me tell you what was considered to be a bright spot of hope: the Internet. The Web was said to have great potential as a tool for change because it's inexpensive and a constantly available resource. Other recent research has revealed that the Internet is just as effective at helping people stick

INSTANT INSPIRATION

"A never-ending goal of mine is to encourage people to make fitness a lifelong, unshakable part of their daily lives, just like breathing. I want to spark an internal fire to chase dreams with unwavering boldness, enthusiasm, and persistence."
—Walker*Defyfate

to diet or fitness plans as face-to-face meetings are.

What does this mean to you and your desire to improve your personal health and fitness—and to make this improvement a lasting change? It means that despite all indications that we live in a time doomed by poor health, we also live in a time that allows us unprecedented access to free and powerful tools for change—it's simply up to you to start using them.

To create a dependable feedback loop that locks out any doubts and makes sure you've achieved "maintainer" status, I've created two action steps that encourage personal responsibility and introduce you to a system of radical accountability.

RADICAL ACCOUNTABILITY ACTION STEPS

Action Step 1: Track Your Progress

An essential part of accountability comes from awareness—remaining conscious of what you're eating and how much you're exercising is critical to helping you stay on track. The problem is, we often rely on our ability to just recall things, but in truth we're really not all that good at remembering details, nor are we good at being unbiased. When you try to remember how many drinks or servings of macaroni and cheese you had at a party, it's pretty much guaranteed that you're going to

underestimate—we have a tendency to want to make ourselves feel good about our choices, which means we also overestimate how good we are at skills in which we're least adept (chances are you really *aren't* that good at dancing the Macarena). Don't worry though, we're all guilty of this; it's just part of being human.

This is why tracking your adherence to a workout or eating plan can be an empowering step toward success. Research has shown that keeping a food journal alone can double weight loss. One study published in the journal *Behavior Therapy* took it a step further by determining that "obsessive-compulsive" self-monitoring was the most effective—this means that the more detailed you are with your records, the better your results.

It's also important to keep track of your progress. When you track your progress either by getting on a scale or by measuring muscle growth, you boost your confidence in your ability to make improvements and to ultimately fulfill your fitness and health goals.

When researchers evaluated a group of people who were successful in making long-term commitments to health and fitness, they found that this thriving group actively kept records of progress, food consumption, and exercise activity. Visit the Resources section in the back of the book for the "Breakthrough Bundle"—a supersized pack of powerful tracking tools that will help you monitor your eating, workouts, and results. You can also create your own BodySpace page to take advantage of the dozens of tracking tools there, including a workout calendar; a log for your body stats, which allows you to generate a progress chart; a strength-training log for workout details; a place to upload progress photos; and several other tools that allow you to get as detailed as you like with your tracking. To create your profile visit www.bodybuilding.com/bodybydesign.

Regardless of how or where you track your details, the most important thing is that you start tracking now—the sooner you wake up to your reality, the quicker you'll experience a truly conscious connection with your health and fitness habits.

INSTANT INSPIRATION

"I love seeing my body changing with each picture that's taken. The way I feel after an intense workout session is second to none!"

—Charlotte*beautifulgrace

Action Step 2: Friendly Feedback

Now that you know how to access measures of personal accountability, it's time to call for reinforcements—to start seeking out what I refer to as friendly feedback. Friendly feedback enlists a community conscience that guarantees there's always someone to answer to for your actions—someone to reach out to for ongoing support and knowledge and constant encouragement.

At this point I'm going to assume that you've followed the action steps in the previous chapters. This means that you've identified individuals or groups of positive influence in your life (or that you've gone outside your immediate circle to establish connections that inspire change) and you've defined and declared your goals. Depending on how you declared your goals—where and with whom—you may have already gained access to friendly feedback. However, this step requires that you be a bit more proactive by ensuring there is a solid system of radical accountability in place, not just the slight chance that it will keep you on track.

Behavioral scientists have shown that the most effective framework of support is one that inspires confidence and trust in you. They've also shown that you are most likely to experience these feelings when a system or network brings accessible knowledge and information, as well as people you can trust, to the table. When I write "trust" here, I'm referring to people with whom you can relate—individuals who started or are currently where you are with your health and fitness levels; with a sense of similarity comes a built-in element of trust and understanding. For example, if we think back to the group of struggling diabetics who connected with other diabetics already in the maintenance phase, the connections they made were life-changing. Those bonds were created quickly and were so effective because the foundation was rooted in the strength of sameness; the newcomers found people who were capable of "challenging their ideas or suggesting simple remedies to problems and always demonstrating a keen interest in their issues."

You may notice that we've crossed back over a bit into the power of social networks and connections. This is because your social network is especially relevant to creating radical accountability that inspires with a bang from the beginning and continues to create long-term motivation. I encourage you to find a network with people who have started where you are. Whether you're 100 pounds overweight, you want to recover your prebaby body, you're disabled, or you want to increase the size of your biceps, you can find a place where people just like you have started and created transformational change.

I have seen people arrive at BodySpace with each of these specific backgrounds—and several hundred thousand more—and connect with others just like them; I think this is an area where "The bigger, the better" rings true—the larger the pool of people, the more likely you are to find someone *you* can connect with. The great thing is, not only are those people ready and willing to grant you access to their path to change, they're there to help keep you accountable. There is a constant chain of feedback going on among visitors to BodySpace—they interact on forums, they comment on personal profiles with words of encouragement, and they track down individuals who inspire them to excel.

Here are a few examples of comments that people have left for me on my own profile page: "Looking absolutely awesome!" "Incredible progress pics." "Hey Kris, thanks for the inspiration and for your program!" "Hi, I wanted to say that you had huge changes in less than four months. How did you lose the fat and gain muscle mass so quickly?" As you can see, it's kind of like having a built-in support team offering nonstop encouragement—this kind of accountability keeps me pumped and motivated!

So your assignment now is to ensure that you have a solid accountability structure in place. You can visit BodySpace to see what we have to offer, but you can also build accountability into your immediate environment by talking to people in your home (family, roommates, etc.) and at your office. Encourage them to check in with you on your progress on a regular basis. Some studies have shown that this kind of support can be more effective if it doesn't initially come from your spouse—I'm not saying this is true for everyone, but some research participants found encouragement from their spouses "annoying" because it

INSTANT INSPIRATION

"I use BodySpace as a constant stream of inspiration and information, through which I'm bound to a community of people like myself struggling for positive change."

—Colin*Cardio Colin

seemed more like nagging or criticism. Certainly if your spouse or significant other has similar goals, you can connect on the shared pursuit of health and fitness (I'll address how to recruit them and others in your life in the next chapter).

My point is, I want you to remember that you are not limited to your immediate surroundings when it comes to creating accountability; you can expand your social network exponentially by creating a BodySpace profile or seek out other networks online and in your region that will give you the structure you need for ultimate success.

"I Now Have the COURAGE to LIVE MY LIFE on My Terms."

"I *wanted* to be more physically active, but I believed that I could not fit it in," says Kassandre Harper-Cotton (BodySpace user name Making_A_Change). "After all, I was a busy wife, mother, student, and worked full-time." Then, suddenly, the "want to" became a "need to," she remembers. "I found myself 185 pounds and extremely dissatisfied with my body and what I was becoming: increasingly self-conscious and lethargic. One day, I even tried to play with my daughter from the couch; I was just exhausted."

She had tried making commitments before, going as far as creating meal plans and workout schedules, but found that she could barely make it through a week; she felt defeated. "When I looked at fitness magazines, I believed that they must have had something that I did not: better genetics, more time, a trainer, a personal chef, an entourage."

"I was ready to change," recalls Kassandre. So she told her husband and a few friends, who seemed supportive but doubtful—they had heard it before. "This time, I was prepared to follow my words with action."

One of her first action steps was to connect with a knowledgeable and supportive network. "I found BodySpace, which became integral to my change. I began blogging and posting progress pictures, which helped me be honest in my efforts, including identifying excuses and logging my small victories," she says. "And, most important, I was able to connect with others who had similar challenges and see how they overcame them."

She began to work out four to six times a week and eat about every three hours, most of the time taking her own meals that she had prepared at home, and eventually she had created new habits. "I have designated times when I eat, and I keep a large container of protein powder and a jar of peanut butter on hand— I look forward to my preplanned meals," she says. "During the day, I am alert and ready to work. I am the type of person I never thought I had the discipline to be."

What remained constant throughout her transformation was her commitment to maintain a high level of accountability. "I

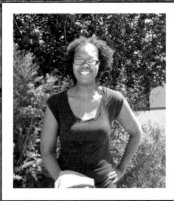

BEFORE

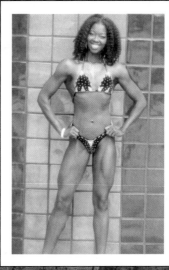

AFTER

made an effort to actively track my progress and to take photos every two to three weeks," she says. "I am proud to say that it shows a slow, sustainable, real-time process." It helped that in addition to the personal accountability she was creating, she was buoyed by a constant support network and ongoing reciprocation of motivation. "It was encouraging to know that while I was on my journey to change my lifestyle, there were others reading my blogs or looking at my progress pictures and feeling motivated, too."

An important change Kassandre made was to overhaul her relationship with food: "As I increased my intensity and frequency in the gym, I began to look at food as fuel; I was eating with a purpose and not absentmindedly," she says. "I was excited by the changes in my body and wanted to see more. I ate to improve the quality of my training, and ultimately my life!"

What started out as a way to get back to her college weight has turned into a full-fledged passion for Kassandre—she has now competed in four figure competitions and is training for the national stage. She's also actively motivating and inspiring others with her experience. "I write motivational articles, and I continue to blog about balancing and integrating healthy habits into one's daily life," she says, noting also that her transformation has opened the eyes of a lot of women in particular. "Women have told me that they no longer fear lifting weights or eating frequently because they could *see* the benefits. It is a humbling feeling to think that something I might have done or said influenced someone to join a gym, compete, or try a little harder."

A renewed sense of confidence has improved nearly every part of Kassandre's life. "I smile a lot more, which makes me more approachable," she says. "I am more likely to initiate and engage someone in a conversation, and as a result, I've grown a beautiful circle of friends. I'm also more assertive and ask for what I need and will voice my opinion—I think getting fit has given me the courage to live my life on my terms. I am happier and healthier."

"Losing Weight Proved to Me That I CAN DO ANYTHING I Want to in Life."

At age 20, Matt Hollingsworth was nearly 300 pounds and wore size 42 pants. Despite excelling in school, he felt his weight held him back in just about every area of his life. "Being overweight affects everything—it creates difficulties and lessens opportunities," he says, acknowledging that his weight left him feeling insecure about approaching girls and creating friendships. "The whole lack of confidence thing definitely limited my experiences. I missed out on the opportunity to really enjoy being an athlete in high school—I swam, but I was pretty terrible at it because of my weight."

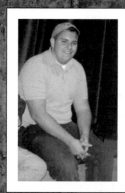

BEFORE

After a few failed attempts at losing weight, Matt felt defeated, but then two things happened to push him into a place of permanent change. "I was at a lake tubing and the tube popped," recalls Matt. "I know it probably wasn't just my weight, but I couldn't stop thinking in my head that it was my nearly 300 pounds that popped it."

Soon after that experience, a friend at work told him if she could combine his personality with a fellow coworker's body, that person would be the "perfect guy." "I know she was trying to partly pay me a compliment, but that just really got to me," says Matt. "There were certainly other experiences with my weight, but those are the most memorable trigger points."

While Matt was motivated to lose weight because of these triggers, he was also motivated to escape a family history of obesity. "Just about everyone on my mom's side of the family is quite overweight," he says. "Growing up, exercise wasn't ever really stressed, and when it came to eating, I would make the healthier choice of not-so-healthy options—I would get a chicken sandwich instead of a hamburger, but I would still get it from McDonald's."

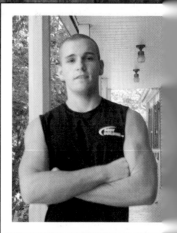

AFTER

Matt had lost some weight before by following a calorie-restricted diet, but not only did he lose fat, he lost valuable muscle as well. "I wanted to look athletic, not skinny and unhealthy," he says. When he was truly ready to commit to a new lifestyle, he turned to BodySpace and searched for people who had a starting point similar to his own who'd also emerged on from their transformation looking fit and muscular. "I spent about two to three hours a night on the computer looking at dozens of profiles," says Matt, whose username is matth0679. "I wrote down things that were successful for them and started combining different aspects of each person's plan. I also started emailing people with questions—these were people I could relate to."

He began running four miles a day and lifting weights in the gym, but his diet was an afterthought and consequently the pounds were slow to budge. "Then, I really started focusing on nutrition—I mean I logged everything," he says. "And I stuck to a specific macronutrient profile every day. It was then that I really began losing."

Matt's motivation took him beyond his original goal to lose 60 pounds—he has now lost more than 100—but he didn't do it all alone. "I told everyone what I was doing," he says. "I figured that if I built enough pressure around me to actually do what I said I would, it would help motivate me to fulfill my goals. I had put my pride on the line."

The solid system of accountability helped him stick to his commitments while completing his senior year of college and preparing for the law school admissions test. Now beginning his first year of law school, Matt views his transformation as something that has set him up for continued success. "I knew that I would not get the respect I could in law school or in the professional world at the weight I was at," he says. "Losing the weight proved to me that I can do anything that I want to in life. One of the hardest things I could ever do is already done, so I can confront almost anything life throws at me."

"I told everyone what I was doing . . . I put my pride on the line."

CHAPTER 6

HOW, Not

What

Just as it's pretty rare for someone to quit smoking "cold turkey," so too is it unrealistic to feel that your health and fitness transformation will happen with the flip of a switch. Sure, the initial transformation trigger will jump-start you on the path to change, but for that change to become habit, you must be patient.

Now, wait! Before you put this book down and pick up the "instant abs" pill instead, I want you to understand something about the choice you have with this life of yours—remember, it's the only one you're going to get! I'm no philosopher, but I am a person who has experienced the incredible advantages a commitment to good health and fitness can bring to your life, so hear me out.

Here's what I see as your two choices:

Option 1: You can spend your days in a body that is something *other*: something that controls you, exhausts you, and quite literally weighs you down—one that you struggle to modify and respect because it's just this clunky, chubby shell you have to drag around. You can continue trying on cosmetic, temporary changes for size as you watch your waistline get bigger and bigger. You can live a life of muted experiences, and you can let the burdens of your body as you age become your identity; if you are diagnosed with diabetes, heart disease, cancer, or any of the other conditions associated with poor diet and lack of exercise, they will begin to define you.

Or, I have another idea for you to consider.

Option 2: You can saddle up the skill you have—that *we all have*—to transform your life through fitness, to create new habits that equal change. You can take control of your life by strategically modifying your behaviors so that they inspire permanent, not fleeting, change. This strategy includes shutting down negative thought patterns that have kept you trapped, identifying an empowering and motivating a network of support, establishing and declaring goals, and monitoring your progress within a reliable framework of accountability (yes, there are a few of the Four Pillars in there). It also includes integrating those strategies on the ground level—pooling them all together and watching them manifest change from the inside out. When you choose this option, you choose to merge the person you are with the person you want to be by uniting your thoughts with your actions, bringing together mind and body. Instead of wishing you could jump up and play in that football game on the beach, go for a run with your daughter and her friends, or help your neighbor move that heavy desk—you can do all of them. Your doubts are no longer your reality; your dreams are!

As we arrive at the final Pillar of Power—the *how,* not the what—I want you to solidify your commitment to your personal transformation. I also want to make sure you have all the tools you need to overcome any obstacles or challenges.

AS EASY AS 1-2-3

Research on creating new habits shows the process as going from gaining knowledge to putting that knowledge into practice to the formation of an "automatic" habit. In other words, you begin by getting the information you need; then you start applying the information to your activities. You continue with this until it becomes automated; like driving your car or brushing your teeth, you just do it. You may have noticed in some of the

BodySpace success stories the acknowledgment of this kind of turning point—when the person was no longer just following a plan but had actually reached a place of certainty and automation. In Part III, you'll find all the information and knowledge you need to create your transformation, but I think it's important for you also to see some additional strategies that have helped others develop lasting change—a little more about *how* they made it happen.

It's been said before that success leaves clues. I've certainly known this to be true, as I've looked to role models throughout my life for direction and inspiration. One study that evaluated people's abilities to either maintain good health habits or relapse into their old ways revealed some pretty important clues. Here are a few of the shared strategies of successful individuals:

1. Be patient.
2. Set small goals.
3. Reduce the amount of food you consume.
4. Stick to a plan; don't be afraid to customize it to your own life.
5. Continue with the plan until it becomes a new pattern.
6. Exercise regularly.

And, so that you will understand too what doesn't work, here are a few of the strategies that unsuccessful individuals have tried:

1. Taking appetite suppressants.
2. Fasting.
3. Seeing diet foods as special foods, different from the foods their family could have.

I want you to keep these lists in mind as you move forward with the Body by Design plan. Though these "do's and don'ts," based on proven success (and failure), are very general, I think they offer excellent starting points for you to consider.

ENSURING YOUR GOALS

Researchers have boiled down the characteristics of habit formation to the finest of details and studied them for revealing evidence. They've taken a look at people who've been able to stick to their goals and asked a lot of questions, such as "Do they just set a goal and sit back and wait for their actions to form new habits?" (I'm sure they actually asked it in more scientific terms, but you get the point.) When they looked at individuals who were trying to commit

INSTANT INSPIRATION

"This site is inspirational, packed with useful info. BodySpace is now starting to connect me to other fitness lovers. As a home-gym trainee, this is the equivalent of hanging out at the gym and library at the same time."

—Mike*BigBlueSquid

to different habits, such as exercising, taking their vitamins, and eating more fruits and vegetables, they realized that those who were the most successful added a little bit of extra insurance, or what the scientists labeled "implementation intentions." These intentions were forms of mental preparation, preprogrammed responses people had established that greatly increased their ability to stick to their goals.

Creating implementation intentions, which I'll refer to as goal insurers, doesn't involve any complicated strategy. In fact, one of the simplest and most effective ensurers is simply to write down the details of the commitment. In an exercise-related study, researchers compared vague statements such as "I'm going to exercise" to the more detailed version "I'm going to work out for sixty minutes at Gold's Gym on Monday at 5:30 A.M." They determined that individuals who wrote down when and where they planned to exercise dramatically increased the behavior.

Three things happen when you fill in the blanks on your commitments like this: you speed up the formation of new habits, you encourage them to become automatic, and you remove the risk of giving in to impulse. Instead of leaving your commitments vulnerable to excuses, you lock your actions into place by taking the simple step of planning ahead. I can say from experience that it's empowering not to feel susceptible to giving into old habits.

You can take proactive measures in many different ways. Since research shows that including the *how* and not just the what, when,

and where is important, I encourage you to take advantage of all the specific program information I've included for you in Part III. It's important to take this information and apply it to circumstances that you may find threatening to your goal commitments. By sticking to the program as I've created it, you help accelerate the formation of automatic habits—there's no guesswork, which positively promotes goal adherence by leaving no room for doubts. This doesn't mean you can't ever get creative with foods and exercises, but until you feel firmly planted in your commitment to good health, I wouldn't stray too far from the plan.

ANTICIPATING OBSTACLES

Another form of goal insurance takes into consideration the scenarios or environments that are most likely to present challenges to your commitment. We've already covered the importance of establishing the details—the what, when, where, and how—but we haven't addressed the inevitable obstacles that will present themselves. The best defense against obstacles is to create an "if-then" game plan.

Researchers have discovered that envisioning "if-then" scenarios is incredibly effective at helping people find an alternative route when roadblocks pop up on the path to their goals. This kind of extra step in preparation helps prevent a lapse in goal adherence. Because you can't always control the forces of influence that exist around you, you have to be diligently proactive, especially as you are forming new habits. In this vulnerable beginning phase, you're more prone to give in to impulsive behaviors based on factors such as mood and environment. When you're prepared, however, you wipe out that risk.

Since behavior can change significantly based on so many variables, it's not as simple as writing off failed attempts at sticking to your goals as being based on a certain personality trait—that is to say, you can't just blame it on the fact that you "have no willpower." (You may recall that willpower doesn't exist in the way that people always thought it did. It's not something you just have or don't have, it's a learned skill, one that often includes simple preparation.) What you can do is consider all those variables and create "if-then" strategies.

My own "if-then" strategies often come into play around the obstacles of lack of time and resources—when I'm slammed with work, I know there's an increased chance that I won't be able to get the food that I need to fuel my body. So instead of thinking "If I'm going to be slammed at work, I'll grab snacks from the vending machine," I prepare, which creates a statement like this: "If I'm going to be slammed at work, I'll eat the grilled chicken and brown rice I prepared at home and packed in a cooler." I'm not exaggerating when I say it's that easy.

There was another time where I had to prepare for two solid days of back-to-back meetings in New York, which, when you need to fuel your body with food every two to three hours, can present a bit of a challenge. So what did I do? I applied the same strategy, because it works and it gives me control over situations that try to threaten my goal commitments. I packed a cooler bag with meals for the entire day, even taking out quick meals to eat during meetings. Several of our BodySpace members talk about taking the same proactive step to control their food options—you'll find this an invaluable tool in helping you create good habits.

You can see that a significant part of developing the skill of goal adherence is knowing how to prepare for challenging situations. As we move into the action steps for this final pillar, I want you to consider what those situations may be for you. They may arise when you're in a certain kind of mood, you're at a party or an event, or you're around a particular person who doesn't support your new habits. Hopefully, you've already made an effort to minimize the influence of unsupportive people, but in this first action step, I'll help you prepare to tackle other potential roadblocks.

GOAL INSURANCE ACTION STEPS

Action Step 1: Create Your "If-Then" Game Plan

Have you determined what, up to this point in your life, has kept you from achieving your goals? Chances are you've identified these obstacles as coming from outside social influences, internal influences (your own thoughts and behavior patterns), or situational influences, or most likely you've discovered that it's a combination of all three. In the Burn and Build Pillar, I addressed how to manage outside social influences (refer back to the action steps on pages 39–42); in the second pillar, I took you through the Prime Time exercise (page 48), which helped you create positive thought patterns. Now I want to give you the best tools for managing situational influences, which are the ones that arise in certain environments, including your own home.

As I've mentioned several times, being able to control your behaviors and actions is a skill, and one that involves a bit of proactive thinking on your part. One of the best ways to describe this ability appeared in a research study, in which the researchers referred to being able to self-regulate as "a skill involving anticipating and cleverness, so that immediate and tempting rewards do not impede progress toward a long-range goal." Basically, planning ahead can be the key to fulfilling your goals.

I've told you about how I use preparation strategies to avoid temptation and keep me on track, and here are some other great examples from our BodySpace members.

"I used to eat M&Ms throughout the day because I would get bored, so instead of having those around I now have grapes, cranberries, or almonds."

—Elijah*SuperMaine

"I have become better at making healthy alternatives to help avoid giving in to cravings. For example, I take my favorite protein powder, extra ice, and blend it to make 'ice cream.' It is very satisfying. There are times too when you just need to ask yourself, 'Is it worth it?' Chances are it is not."

—Kassandre*Making_A_Change

"Having a scale will help push you over the cravings and weaknesses. Since the scale doesn't lie you can't cheat without it showing it to you."

—Dustin*GOGOGTO

"Don't have any junk foods in the house. You are less likely to go out for ice cream or a chocolate bar than you are to just reach in the fridge or cupboard for it."

—Errol*Captain Ahab

"If you don't plan, you will lose your way and keep justifying eating foods and meals that will set you up to fail— you must plan! I plan for my cheat meals as well. I eat clean for eight to eleven days before, and I make my cheat meals last for only forty minutes—no more. When I'm done, I'm done. Then it's back to eight to eleven more days of healthy eating."

—Ed*oldsuperman

In these examples, you can see an awareness of the situations that may present temptation—and the steps these individuals have taken to ensure that they don't derail their progress. These are people who have been extremely successful in transforming their lives with fitness; they no longer accept excuses for living a life that's inconsistent with achieving their goals.

To create your own "If-Then" Game Plan, think about areas in your life that lead to situational excuses. Begin to consider how you can turn a negative into a positive. Instead of saying "I don't have time to exercise," say, "If I wake up thirty minutes earlier in the morning and watch fifteen minutes less TV at night, I will have forty-five minutes for exercise." Write down five situations that present weaknesses for you, and then create the positive, proactive response that will help you refuse to accept excuses any longer.

Step 2: Create Collaborative Motivation

First off, congratulations for making it to the final step in the Pillars of Power. If you've followed all the steps up to this point, I know you have ignited a true fire in your motivation and you're on the path to lasting change. Since you've already done all that hard work, this last step will require a little less effort on your part.

Hopefully, you've already taken steps to connect with a solid social network that will provide you with support and ongoing accountability, but I want to make sure you haven't completely overlooked those closest to you.

As you're about to discover the specifics of the Body by Design plan, I want you to think about anyone in your life whom you might want to recruit to do it with you. I'm not talking specifically about your significant other (although you can certainly include him or her) but rather your friends—even the ones you've essentially eliminated from your circle of influence. Though this may sound strange, it's actually very strategic.

When you recruit three friends to participate in the transformation with you, you actually greatly increase your chances of creating long-term adherence to your new health habits—at least according to one study published in the *Journal of Consulting and Clinical Psychology*. Researchers determined that when people started a weight-loss program with three friends, 95 percent of them were successful with the program, and nearly 70 percent of participants were able to maintain their habits in the long term. This means that adding an extra layer of support can further strengthen your foundation for success.

I also encourage you to reach out to those you previously identified as detractors. Though I wouldn't have recommended doing this earlier in the book, the heightened level of awareness you now have should give you a brand-new sense of confidence in your commitments. Invite those people to join you as you begin your transformation. Bringing them on board can only further strengthen your ultimate purpose; plus, you'll officially have enlisted yourself as a messenger of the fitness movement of Body by Design.

"Food Was My ADDICTION."

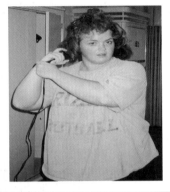

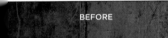

BEFORE

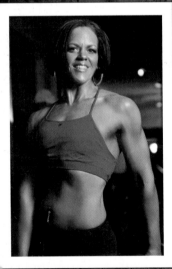

AFTER

"I had reached my all-time low," recalls Amy Barnes. "I was living in a battered women's shelter; I had no job, no home, and no car, and I weighed 490 pounds with a BMI of 52 percent!"

Barnes, who goes by 325Down on BodySpace, a nod to her more than 300-pound weight loss, says her story is one that many women can relate to. "I found myself in an abusive relationship, and I found solace in the food that I ate," she says. "I felt that the only thing I had control over in my life was the food I put in my mouth; food was my addiction, just as alcohol to an alcoholic."

As the mother of two boys, Barnes knew she had to make a revolutionary life change. "I did not want my boys to grow up being embarrassed of me or, worse, losing their mom to an obesity-related health issue—I hated myself."

She tried every fad diet on the market and every over-the-counter and prescription weight-loss pill she could find. "I bought into every quick fix and infomercial that told me I was guaranteed to lose weight 'or my money back.' I was willing to try anything." Then she discovered the truth: "Despite what marketers tell you, there are no quick fixes when it comes to adopting a healthy lifestyle."

Barnes reflects back on how living a healthy life became a lifestyle—when working out and eating healthfully became "like brushing my teeth." Here she shares her top five strategies for success:

1. **SEEK SOCIAL SUPPORT.** "I was an emotional eater, so the things that caused stress or negative emotions, I removed from my life—this included people. If there were people in my life who were not supportive or who made me feel bad about myself, I knew those influences didn't have my best interest at heart. I instead surrounded myself with like-minded people, people dedicated to living and leading a healthy life. I wanted to be around people who would motivate me to be better for myself. On BodySpace, I found people all striving for the same thing I was—even though each person had

a different starting point, we all were striving to make and change our bodies."

2. **SET GOALS.** "First, make the commitment to finally do something for yourself—no excuses. Every day, find a time when you will put yourself first—this helps create full commitment. Second, set and identify reasonable goals and expectations for yourself; set weekly, monthly, and yearly goals. I always say that every journey needs a map, and setting out to change your lifestyle is no exception!"

3. **BE ACCOUNTABLE.** "The key to maintaining successful habits is to keep monitoring your progress and not to lose accountability to yourself. In a world full of temptations, it's easy to slip back into bad habits if you don't stay focused on why you made the changes in the first place. The biggest goal here is to be the best you can be for yourself. I can reflect back on many changes I made in my life, and they all required striving to be something better than I was at that moment."

4. **THINK DIFFERENTLY ABOUT EATING.** "I never called it a diet because in the past, all of the other 'diets' never worked for me. Without changing how you eat and how you think about food, you will never lose the weight. When I finally stopped letting food control me and I was able to take control over food and how I felt about it, the weight dropped off—and all without calling it a diet."

5. **EXERCISE.** "When first starting out, I walked—that was really all my body could handle, along with light resistance training. As the weight started to drop, I continued to lift weights, which improved tone, and increased muscle, which in turn boosted my metabolism and contributed to my weight loss. I also became a huge advocate of group classes. The time goes fast, there is an instructor to push you, and, with others in the class, you make friends who have similar interests to yours."

Her transformation also inspired a career overhaul. "I quit my job in corporate America to help other people find the peace and happiness that I had found through a healthier lifestyle," she says with pride. "I started my own fitness company, and now I get to help people write their own stories—I am healthy, happy, and now get to spend my life motivating others."

From Hurt, Depressed, and Skinny to HEALED, JOYFUL, and Muscular

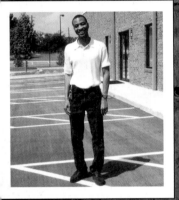

BEFORE

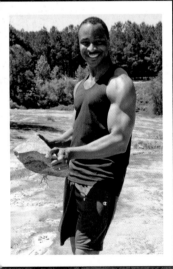

AFTER

"When I started my transformation journey, it seemed like everything in my life was falling apart," says Ricky Howell. "I was struggling financially, and my marriage of eleven years had just ended in divorce. When you're hurting emotionally, it becomes extremely difficult to find the motivation you need to go forward and believe that things will get better."

Ricky didn't have a choice, though—he was granted custody of his two children and had to pull his life together; he decided to start with an area where he knew he could regain some control: his health. "I wasn't taking very good care of myself. I was working a lot of hours, skipping meals, eating fast foods, and not getting quality rest," he says. "I knew if things didn't change that I would be putting my health and long-term well-being at risk."

With his personal drive running at full speed, Ricky initially kept his fitness goals to himself and began working out and doing research. Then his friends started to notice the changes to his body. "They started asking questions," he says. "I had friends wanting to work out and get healthy because of my transformation."

He wasn't entirely alone during this process, though—in fact, he had access to a support system of hundreds of thousands of people. "BodySpace is my social support group—it's a great tool because you have the opportunity to communicate with other fitness-minded people from around the world," says Ricky, who's known as kratoscomm there. "You can learn from others who have more experience than you, receive motivation, and become a source of inspiration and encouragement to others who are just starting their journey."

Though Ricky says he initially stumbled on BodySpace because it was linked to the site where he did nutrition and workout research, once he discovered it, it became essential to his progress. "BodySpace quickly became a source of inspiration—seeing the profiles and reading the background stories of how some of the members got started on their road to fitness gave me encouragement," he says. "I filled in my personal and background information, progress pictures, body stats, and goals. Soon after that I began communicating and finding members who were willing to answer questions and provide great advice on how to achieve my fitness goals."

Part of the lesson Ricky learned from connecting to a social network is that the little effort you put in up front can pay off in dividends. "You need positive people who support your fitness goals, you need someone or a support group that you can learn from and be accountable to, and you need to share your story so that others can be inspired and motivated," he says. "Oftentimes we feel that our transformation is just for us, but it's also for other people—there is someone who can identify with your life experience, and they need to know that if you can overcome your challenges and reach your goals, then they can do the same. I have combined these tools to help create an environment that allows me to flourish in my fitness pursuits. A few years ago, I could not imagine that I could have gone from being hurt, depressed, and skinny to healed, joyful, and muscular."

Ricky also takes pride in how his habits have impacted his family and friends. "I have recently remarried, and now my wife is interested in weight training due to my example," he notes. "Since I live a healthy lifestyle, my kids understand the importance of healthy eating and exercise, and my friends have become interested in fitness."

Here Ricky shares some motivational tips for staying on track.

1. Don't be intimidated by others who are more advanced in their development than you—everyone starts from somewhere.
2. Stay consistent with your diet and training. If you stumble due to discouragement or lack of results, get back up and try again.
3. Don't focus on others and how fast they are reaching their fitness goals. Learn to run your race; everyone's journey is different.
4. You have to believe in your heart that you're a winner and that you can reach your goal.

> "A few years ago, I could not imagine that I could have gone from being hurt, depressed, and skinny to healed, joyful, and muscular."

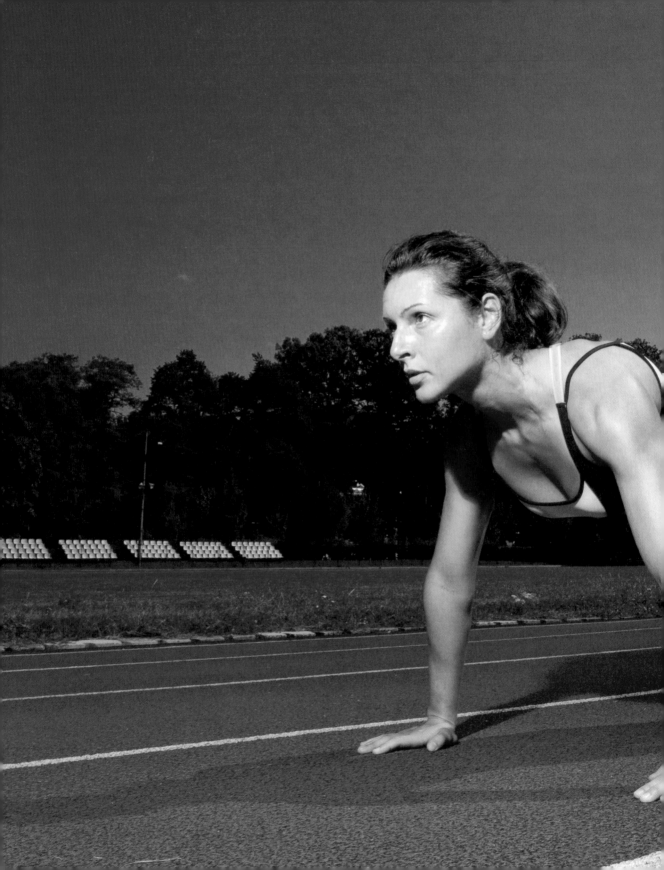

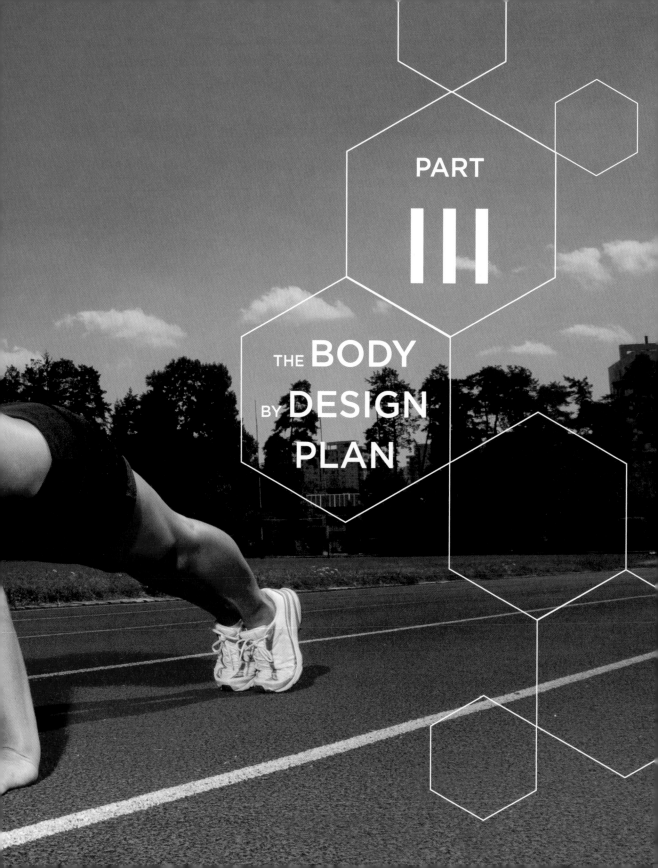

PART

III

THE BODY
BY DESIGN
PLAN

CHAPTER 7

The Body by Design

WORKOUT PLAN

Of course, all the motivation in the world won't do you a bit of good if you don't have a strong fitness plan to follow. That's what this section of the book is about: I'll give you a clear, simple, and effective plan to follow in the gym to help you reach your goals, no matter if you want to gain muscle, lose fat, or just drop a clothing size. It doesn't matter if you're a gym rat or if you're just starting out with your fitness journey. With this twelve-week plan, you can transform your body.

The great thing about the Body by Design plan is that it's tested. Thousands upon thousands of people have put these principles into action—and you've met many of them already in the pages of this book. But the stories you've heard so far are just a fraction of the amazing transformations I've witnessed firsthand. And don't think I've only been watching from the sidelines. In addition to coaching others, I have gone through my own transformation process myself more times than I can count. (I have reached a level of fitness where eating healthfully and strength training are my lifestyle, so my "transformations" are less lifestyle overhauls than they are studies of my own body and how I can truly maximize its performance and development.) Trying different types of nutrition and workout strategies has allowed me to become a better coach for you—and it's the reason why I can now present you with what works best.

The incredible thing is that whenever I have transformed my body, I have transformed my life—inevitably, conquering the physical and mental challenges of a transformation carries over into many other areas of my life. In fact, recommitting to a body transformation literally seems to open doors for me. I find it no coincidence that when I completed my first transformation, I went from working in a wood furniture warehouse to studying international health and sports therapy. After my second transformation, I found myself traveling the Caribbean as a massage therapist on cruise liners; after the third, running my own fitness center in Sydney, Australia; after the fourth, becoming a writer and photographer for the leading health magazines in Los Angeles, California; and after the fifth, becoming editor in chief of Bodybuilding.com. I recently completed another transformation. The result? My best physical transformation yet—and I get the privilege of writing this book for you to create your own journey.

The question is, when you commit to your transformation, *what doors are going to open for you?* Will you become a better parent because of your newfound energy, a better coworker because of your confidence, a better spouse because your energy, confidence, *and* appearance have made you more attractive to your partner? Or maybe you'll become all of those things and more. One thing's for sure, though: you and everyone who loves you will reap the benefits of your commitment to good health and longevity.

INSTANT INSPIRATION

"I love being able to sculpt my physique through hard work. Lifting weights is a spiritual experience for me and gets me through to the other side of any situation I am dealing with."

—Ava*AvaCowan

When you follow this program, the physical transformation you will experience will be just the tip of the iceberg; it will be the gateway to taking control of your life and creating positive changes in many different areas. Let me tell you a little more about why strength training is the number one method for changing your body and your life.

THE CASE FOR WEIGHTS

There are many names for it—strength training, weight training, resistance training, pumping iron, and bodybuilding are a few that come to mind. In the end, what you call it doesn't matter; that you *do* it does. The activity is the same regardless of how you label it—either way you're going to lift some weights. You can accomplish incredible benefits with weights that you simply can't with any other form of exercise, which is why I want to quickly clear up a few misconceptions about strength training.

Maybe you have never really tried strength training before. It can be intimidating. Throughout my years as a trainer, writer, and editor, one of my most difficult struggles has been to educate people—in particular, women—about the importance of strength training. The majority of women steer clear of the weights area for fear of looking bulky or developing a "manly" appearance.

That isn't going to happen—at least not on the Body by Design program.

Women simply don't have the genetics or testosterone present to add muscle that rapidly or dramatically. Even by following the carefully crafted strength-building program in this book, a woman will not get an overly muscled physique. I always say that just because you start a new job at a company as the receptionist, it doesn't necessarily mean you will become the CEO overnight. Just as singing in the shower won't make you sound like Diana Ross or Bono. The same goes for weight training: Arnold's arms won't sprout out of you simply because you become a regular in the weights area at the gym.

When you start training regularly with weights, your muscles develop, become denser, and burn more calories all day and night. Though cardio is a great way to assist in fat loss, it burns fat only while you're performing the exercise, not around the clock. Lifting weights and adding lean muscle, on the other hand, turns your body into a full-time calorie-burning machine. If you were to add just 5 pounds of muscle to your frame, you could burn an additional 250 to 300 calories per day—that's a whole meal for some people! As I sit here writing this in a coffee shop, I am happy with my lean and muscular body fat

INSTANT INSPIRATION

"Being just skinny doesn't look good after 30; it translates into saggy butt and arms with a jiggle. You *can* have a great body [and discover] that it's empowering to be physically strong."

—Fern*MsFitFern

levels and I know that I can grab a banana muffin from the counter if I want to because my muscle density will burn it off for me—I don't have to rely on the "makeup" cardio I see so many others turning to. Too often I find myself in the lonely weights area watching people as they fill up the rows of cardio machines and move frantically about; I shake my head and think to myself, "If only they knew the real key to fat loss."

You've probably heard the phrase "Muscle weighs more than fat" before, which might lead you to believe that adding muscle is going to make you a heavier, bulkier person. First off, muscle is not heavier than fat—a pound of muscle is equal to a pound of fat. Muscle is more compact than fat, though, which means it takes up less space, so the more muscle you add to your body, the more compact and lean you will look; it has a tightening effect. And unless you are following a specific eating plan to gain weight and bulk up, you will never achieve a bulky appearance, so you don't have to worry about that happening.

That being said, I want to point out that it is likely that men will add more muscle on this program. Since guys have higher testosterone levels, they are genetically more capable of adding muscle. When a correctly designed weight-training program—that is, one that places the necessarily amount of stress on the muscles, stimulating growth—is followed, men's bodies will respond by adding muscle to their frames. Keep in mind that you can have the goal of building muscle and burning fat; adding muscle will promote fat burning. The key here is to make sure that you fuel your body frequently and appropriately, which is why I want you to make sure you read all about nutrition in the next chapter.

Strength training has a long list of benefits. The amazing thing is that these benefits aren't limited to just one type of person; lifting weights can produce the same type of gains for men and women, both young and old. Though there are several other ways strength training can help improve your life, here are some of the top research-supported reasons for picking up those weights today:

➤ You'll increase your daily calories burned (I already pointed this out, but I think it's worth repeating).

➤ You will reduce your risk of developing high blood pressure, heart disease, cancer, and obesity.

➤ You'll feel happier and help ward off depression.

➤ You'll keep your brain sharp (research that appeared in Brain and Cognition revealed that just thirty minutes of exercise can boost brain performance).

➤ You will improve your bone density and reduce osteoarthritis pain.

➤ You'll help prevent diabetes by improving your insulin response.

➤ You will sleep better.

➤ You'll boost your longevity.

➤ You'll strengthen your body and help prevent injury.

➤ You will improve your balance.

I'd say that's a pretty strong case for strength training, but it doesn't include my number one reason for lifting weights: increased energy. My energy is boosted for the entire day after a workout—once you get started, you'll discover that it's an addictive energy you can't wait to tap into! I always laugh to myself when people say they're too tired to work out—well, if I didn't exercise on a regular basis, I wouldn't have the energy either. This is energy you can use to fuel transformations in other areas of your life, including in your career. Research has shown that exercising during the workday can increase productivity—if you miss a morning workout, eat a quick lunch at your desk and head to the gym; you'll re-

turn invigorated and ready to make things happen.

Now that you're primed with plenty of reasons to get started with strength training, let's get to the details of the plan.

YOUR TRAINING SCHEDULE

You will be working out with weights only three days of the week. I recommend you train one day, take the following day off to rest and recover your trained muscles, then train again on the next day. So the basic Body by Design plan has your strength-training workouts on Monday, Wednesday, and Friday so you can take the weekend off from the gym. If you need to shift the workout days to fit your schedule, just be sure to structure it so you have two days in a row off from weights at some point.

Be sure to stick to no more than three workouts in a week—don't add in extra strength-training sessions, because they will actually *slow down* your progress, not accelerate it. A lot of people believe that more is better and end up adding in workouts, but this is definitely not the best strategy when trying to shape your body.

I've had people who've followed my programs ask why they haven't gotten the results my other clients have. In most cases, I've discovered that they've added more workout days, thinking they will get better re-

INSTANT INSPIRATION

"I was sick with asthma and hospitalized a lot as a kid and I love the feeling of being healthy and strong now. I want to be in good shape throughout my life and there are no magical pills to stay fit so I keep working hard."

—Laura*ChickenTuna

sults. The problem with this is that your body *needs* the rest days—this is the time when your muscles recover and rebuild. I have designed your workouts with a focus on the quality of the workout over the quantity—trust that they will create the change you desire in your body.

When it comes down to it, you will get your desired body through rest, recovery, and nutrition. In the gym, your job is to stimulate stress on your muscles so they require rest; then you must provide your body with the proper fuel (food) so that it can generate progress and results. When you overtrain and overstress your body, the side effects can include progressive loss of strength, tiredness, loss of appetite, disrupted sleep, loss of motivation, and irritability. For this reason, your workouts should take no longer than one hour at the absolute maximum, and rest times between every set should be no longer than one minute. If you can train much longer than the times I have recommended, I suggest you try to up the intensity—if you're training the right way, you shouldn't be able to train for hours on end.

WHEN FAILURE IS A GOOD THING

All repetitions should be completed to absolute failure on every exercise. When I say "failure," I mean you push your muscles to the point at which you just can't do another rep. For example, if you're required to do twelve repetitions of an exercise, the last three or four should be a real struggle, so much so that you couldn't do another rep even if you wanted to. The first eight or nine reps don't do anything to shape your physique at all; it's the last few that create change in your body. If you only go through the motions and don't challenge yourself, expect that lackluster effort to be reflected back at you in the mirror. I have seen it with my very own eyes—people who go to the gym for years, sometimes even with a personal trainer, and they end up looking exactly the same because they do what they have always done, so they get what they have always got.

When you train to failure, you create microscopic tears in your muscle fibers, which is why you experience soreness. This is not to be confused with pushing yourself to the point of extreme pain and injury. The idea is that these small tears will create soreness, not injury; there's a big difference between the two. Once you have broken your muscle fibers down, your body requires rest and protein to repair the tears (in the next chapter, I'll share with you the best forms of protein and also some suggestions for supplements that will help minimize soreness). The muscle will then respond by growing in size and density in preparation for the likelihood of a larger stress being placed upon it. The most important thing to remember when it comes to your strength-training sessions: don't hold back in your workouts, and your results won't hide from you.

To ensure you get the most out of your workouts, you must pay attention to proper weight selection. You want to be sure to perform the exercises with an amount of weight that will put your muscles under the right amount of stress. Guys, don't train with your ego, and ladies, you are stronger than you think—and please remember that challenging your muscles does not mean bulking them up. The key is to use a weight that allows you to maintain proper form (study the images that accompany the exercises for a demonstration of proper form). Here's an easy way to test what weight you should be using: if you find yourself reaching failure at three or more reps higher than the required amount, increase the weight; if you find that you stop three or more reps short of the required number, lighten the load a little.

THE IMPORTANCE OF CARDIO TRAINING

I recommend you do cardio training every day, which includes your strength-training days. On your strength-training days, I want you to do 20 minutes of cardio in the morning, immediately following breakfast. It can be a brisk walk, a jog, or a session on a cardio machine in your gym. On your nontraining days, I would like you to do cardio immediately following breakfast and again at some point in the afternoon or evening. It doesn't really matter what time you do it, but make sure you do it at least five hours after your first cardio session to better help spike your metabolism.

Cardio should be performed at a moderate intensity. I don't want you to just go for a stroll, but I don't want you doing an all-out sprint. You should walk with the intention to work up a good sweat and increase your heart rate to the point where you're just on the verge of feeling out of breath. I like to use the "talk test" as my intensity meter—if I can still talk to someone without gasping for air, I'm at the perfect pace. You'll basically be walking as fast as you can without needing to break into a jog—this is the perfect intensity for burning fat and not muscle. If you want to use a more scientific method to get your ideal heart-rate zone for fat burning, you can use this simple formula: subtract your age from 220 (the maximum heart rate) and then calculate 60 to 70 percent of this number. For example, if you are 35, it would look like this:

220 (maximum heart rate) – 35 (age) = 185 (maximum heart rate for age); 60–70 percent of 185 = 111 – 129 (target heart rate zone for age)

If you perform cardio at a snail's pace, your

heart rate will not increase enough to burn fat for energy and you will be trying to figure out why you're not experiencing maximum results. On the other hand, if you perform cardio too intensely, you risk burning muscle, which will also impede your progress. So for the purposes of this program, aim for the moderate pace I described. Also, make sure that your intensity is consistent for the whole duration; don't stop or slow down. It takes time for the body to use fat as energy, so if you decide to slow down or stop, you will slow down or stop your results.

Cardio is to be performed for a maximum of 30 minutes—we'll start with just 20 minutes, then increase it to 25 in the second phase, then max out at 30 in phase three. Any longer than this, and you run the risk of slowing your metabolism and burning muscle. I've witnessed thousands of transformations and tested dozens of scenarios on myself, and I've discovered that a maximum of 30 minutes of moderate cardio is the perfect amount for maintaining muscle and burning fat.

So this is how your weeks will look:

MON	TUES	WED	THURS	FRI	SAT	SUN
A.M. Cardio + Strength Workout	A.M. Cardio + P.M. Cardio	A.M. Cardio + Strength Workout	A.M. Cardio + P.M. Cardio	A.M. Cardio + Strength Workout	A.M. Cardio + P.M. Cardio	A.M. Cardio + P.M. Cardio

➤ Strength training with weights three days a week

➤ 20 to 30 minutes of cardio every morning, with another session in the afternoon or evening on your non-strength-training days

➤ No more than 60 minutes in the gym, three times per week

Sounds pretty doable, right? It is. And though the amount of time you spend in the gym each week will be constant, what you do while you're there will change periodically, so your body will continually be working harder to keep up. Now let me tell you about the three different training phases of the Body by Design plan.

The BODY BY DESIGN Workouts

There are three different training phases: the Fundamental Phase, the Momentum Phase, and the DTP Phase. These phases place a progressive amount of stress on your muscles, which will result in an extremely significant change in your appearance; all you have to do is apply it. Remember, this is just the *information* you need—your motivation and drive should be fully ignited by the action steps you applied in the Pillars of Power chapters; be sure to check out Chapters 3 through 6 if you haven't already done so.

Regardless of your environment, whether you have long work hours, a certain disability, or lack of energy or time, the degree of your success ultimately comes down to how successful you've been in tapping into your mental drive; if your mind is motivated, focused, and prepared, your body will follow. The common theme I've witnessed in most BodySpace transformations is that establishing control over the mental environment is the essential first step—so don't skip it!

You've already established your goals in the action steps from Chapter 4, which means you've taken a significant step toward success. Thus far in this chapter, I've given you a substantial overview of the plan, but I haven't gotten to what I consider to be the most critical part of the exercise section: the workout trackers. Let's just say that if the exercise portion of this book caught fire and all you were left with was the trackers, you could complete the entire twelve-week plan. I'm not saying that the rest of the information isn't valuable; I've just made an extra effort to make sure the trackers further fortify your commitments to the plan. In this chapter, I'll take you through a sample week for each of the three phases. You will follow the Fundamental Phase for five weeks, the Momentum Phase for four weeks, and the DTP Phase for three weeks.

In the Resources section on page 191, you will find blank trackers you can fill in yourself. You can copy those and take them to the gym with you, buy a notebook to record the information about your workout, or visit the website for this book (www.bodybuilding.com/bodybydesign) to find customizable online trackers that will guide you through the entire twelve-week program. When you visit the link, simply follow the instructions you see there and your online tracker will

INSTANT INSPIRATION

"Besides using weights to rebound from illness and injuries, I just love doing it. It's the ultimate rush for me to feel stronger, watching my weights move up and watching my appearance change."

—Chad*thenaturaloneky1

automatically be populated with the Body by Design workout program. Logging your training sessions is essential, because it compels honesty and gives you concrete markers of progress—like notches of growth, each representing one step closer to achieving your goals.

Remember that the weight levels used in the handwritten trackers in this chapter are just for demonstration purposes; you should customize the weights to suit your own fitness level (refer back to page 91 for instructions on weight selection). When you're ready to start your workout you'll find the exercises instructions and images in the Exercise Database on page 147.

Be sure to also check out the Transformation Triggers near the conclusion of each phase—these are two quick tips that will give you a mental and physical edge as you begin each phase. Let's get to a brief overview of each of the phases and how they'll carry you through to a truly amazing transformation.

1. THE FUNDAMENTAL PHASE (WEEKS 1–5)

This crucial first phase is designed to prepare your body for radical transformation. It is the perfect starting point for anyone, regardless of your experience with weights—the exercises are basic but powerful, and you will find them clearly demonstrated in the descriptions and accompanying images in the Exercise Database starting on page 147. No matter what your current physical shape, the Fundamental Phase will create the base on which phenomenal results can build.

We'll begin with isolation movements, which focus primarily on working a single muscle to prefatigue; then we will add in a

BREATHE RIGHT

Always be sure to maintain your breathing during each and every rep. Many beginners hold their breath while training, which doesn't allow sufficient oxygen to get to the muscles, and performance and progress are thereby hindered. On the positive portion (the lifting part) of the rep, exhale; on the negative (the return portion), inhale. This will ensure that your muscles have plenty of oxygen to function at their best and keep your body in sync with the movements you're performing, giving you an extra bit of momentum.

SET UP FOR SUCCESS

WARM-UP SET: A trial set of the exercise or exercises you're about to perform; usually done with lighter weights with the purpose of warming up the muscles and joints.

WORKING SETS: The sets that follow your warm-up set. These are the sets that require you to use enough weight to allow you to reach absolute failure at the intended amount of repetitions. If the goal set by the Body by Design program is to reach twelve repetitions but you can do sixteen, you need to increase the weight so you can only just manage about twelve. Conversely, if you can do only eight reps, you need to decrease the load.

compound, or multimuscle, movement that uses several assisting muscles. When you combine these types of exercises, you ensure that the muscle is worked to full capacity and you create distinct development from one muscle to the next—this is key to developing a toned appearance. Keep in mind, though, that at this stage it will be unlikely to see the development if you have a layer of fat covering the muscle. Don't worry, there is work going on under there that will reveal itself in just a short matter of time. I promise!

The Fundamental Phase will also prepare your muscles, tendons, and ligaments for the heavier and more intense training of the second phase. During this first phase, you will perform three sets of each exercise. As you begin the program, I want you to maintain proper focus on form, breathing, and your level of intention: commit yourself to getting the most out of every minute you spend working out. When you establish good

habits like this early on, you lower the likelihood of injury and maximize your body's ability to make progress and achieve stunning results.

The Fundamental Phase should be followed exactly as it is structured for a total of five weeks. Be sure to challenge yourself to train harder each week, each day, and through each set—that way your body will not adapt to the exercises and will continue to change shape. The key to continually creating a challenge for your body is to accurately track the details of your workouts—if you rely just on what "feels challenging" on a particular day, you risk undermining your body's true potential simply because your mood or energy may be different.

Since the first phase is the longest of all three phases at five weeks, I want you to consider this as a five-week challenge before moving on to the second phase. That way you focus on achievable, smaller goals set up within

TRANSFORMATION TRIGGERS—PHASE ONE

MIND-SET MOTIVATION

Use visualization techniques on the way to the gym or as you are warming up prior to starting your workout. Visualize the body you aspire to in your mind and see yourself existing in your daily life with this body—picking up your kids with strength instead of back pain, slipping into your favorite jeans to discover that they fit perfectly, feeling excited about a pool party instead of dreading the moment when someone says, "Come on, take off your shirt and jump in the water!" Prepping your mind with these positive images will help you feel motivated from the moment you set foot in the gym.

PHYSICAL PREPARATION

Starting in the Fundamental Phase, I recommend creating a good warm-up habit. Before you start with your weight training session, jump on a cardio machine for five minutes, or at the very least walk around the block. This will help warm up your muscles and prepare them for activation. Plus, a warm-up helps lower the likelihood of injury and lubricates your joints. To further activate your muscles prior to your working sets, perform one to three warm-up sets of each exercise— this will really help get your blood flowing, especially if your body feels stiff and tired.

the larger goal of your transformation—this will keep your motivation fully charged.

Planning for Repeat Progress

Starting with this first phase, I want you to establish a solid habit of tracking your workouts. When you track your workouts from the very beginning, you set the foundation for consistent progress by creating ongoing connections with your body and its abilities; each of these connections provides an invaluable springboard that will propel your results forward again and again. You can find the blank template for the Fundamental Phase in the Resources section. You will repeat this same plan for five weeks (35 days), so be sure to make enough copies.

In the blank trackers on pages 193–202, you'll notice that I had to fill in only the weights used and the actual number of reps I completed. The target reps are the number you should be aiming for, but if you fall short or long of the goal, write it down and make adjustments next time—this, again, is why it's essential to keep accurate and detailed logs of your workouts.

BODY BY DESIGN SAMPLE FUNDAMENTAL PHASE WORKOUT TRACKER

Phase 1, Day 1: Back, Upper Traps, & Biceps

DAY 1

Date: 1/10
Day __1__ of 35

A.M. Cardio (20 minutes) ☒

EXERCISE	SET 1: TR	WEIGHT/ AR	SET 2: TR	WEIGHT/ AR	SET 3: TR	WEIGHT/ AR	SET 4: TR	WEIGHT/ AR
Lateral Pulldowns	15	50 lbs/15	15	50 lbs/15	15	50 lbs/15		
Seated Cable Rows	15	60 lbs/15	15	60 lbs/15	15	60 lbs/15		
Dumbbell Shrugs	15	20 lbs/15	15	40 lbs/15	15	40 lbs/15		
Hyperextensions	12	0/20	12	0/20	12	0/20		
Biceps Cable Curls	15	40 lbs/15	15	40 lbs/15	15	40 lbs/15	15	40 lbs/15
Concentration Curls	15	30 lbs/15	15	30 lbs/15	15	30 lbs/15	15	30 lbs/15

Phase 1, Day 2: Cardio and Upper Abs

DAY 2

Date: 1/11
Day __2__ of 35

A.M. Cardio (20 minutes) ☒
P.M. Cardio (20 minutes) ☒

EXERCISE	SET 1: TR	AR	SET 2: TR	AR	SET 3: TR	AR	SET 4: TR	AR
Abdominal Crunches	20	20	20	20	20	20		

Phase 1, Day 3: Chest and Triceps

DAY 3

Date: 1/12
Day __3__ of 35

A.M. Cardio (20 minutes) ☒

EXERCISE	SET 1: TR	WEIGHT/ AR	SET 2: TR	WEIGHT/ AR	SET 3: TR	WEIGHT/ AR	SET 4: TR	WEIGHT/ AR
Dumbbell Flyes	15	20 lbs/15	15	20 lbs/15	15	20 lbs/15		
Dumbbell Bench Press	15	30 lbs/15	15	30 lbs/15	15	30 lbs/15		
Incline Dumbbell Flyes	15	20 lbs/15	15	20 lbs/15	15	20 lbs/15		
Triceps Cable Extensions	15	60 lbs/15	15	60 lbs/15	15	60 lbs/15		
Bench Dips	15	0 lbs/15	15	0 lbs/15	15	0 lbs/15		
Overhead Triceps Cable Extensions	15	50 lbs/15	15	50 lbs/15	15	50 lbs/15		

NOTES

Proud of myself for getting to the gym—first time in awhile! Started out too light on D.B. Shrugs—start at 40 next time. Didn't get to failure until 20 reps on hyperextensions—add 10lb. weight next week. Not as sore as I thought I would be on Day 2 . . . maybe the hot bath helped.

Phase 1, Day 4: Cardio and Lower Abdominals

DAY 4

Date: 1/13
Day __4__ of 28

A.M. Cardio (20 minutes) ☒
P.M. Cardio (20 minutes) ☒

EXERCISE	SET 1: TR	AR	SET 2: TR	AR	SET 3: TR	AR	SET 4: TR	AR
Lying Leg Raises	20	20	20	20	20	20		

Phase 1, Day 5: Shoulders and Legs

DAY 5

Date: 1/14
Day __5__ of 35

A.M. Cardio (20 minutes) ☒

EXERCISE	SET 1: TR	WEIGHT/ AR	SET 2: TR	WEIGHT/ AR	SET 3: TR	WEIGHT/ AR	SET 4: TR	WEIGHT/ AR
Side Dumbbell Raises	15	20 lbs/15	15	20 lbs/15	15	20 lbs/15		
Front Dumbbell Raises	15	20 lbs/15	15	20 lbs/15	15	20 lbs/15		
Dumbbell Shoulder Press	15	30 lbs/15	15	30 lbs/15	15	30 lbs/15		
Leg Extensions	20	90 lbs/20	20	90 lbs/20	20	90 lbs/15		
Lying Leg Curls	15	50 lbs/15	15	50 lbs/15	15	50 lbs/15		
Leg Press	15	170 lbs/15	15	170 lbs/15	15	170 lbs/15		
Standing Calf Raises	15	80 lbs/15	15	80 lbs/15	15	80 lbs/15		

Phase 1, Day 6: Cardio

DAY 6

Date: 1/15
Day __6__ of 35

A.M. Cardio (20 minutes) ☒
P.M. Cardio (20 minutes) ☒

Phase 1, Day 7: Cardio

DAY 7

Date: 1/16
Day __7__ of 35

A.M. Cardio (20 minutes) ☒
P.M. Cardio (20 minutes) ☒

NOTES

_____
_____
_____
_____
_____

Key: TR=Target Reps; AR=Actual Reps

2. THE MOMENTUM PHASE (WEEKS 6-9)

Throughout the Fundamental Phase, your tendons, ligaments, muscles, and mind have been given a jump start, and you're now prepared for the increased intensity that will be used throughout phase two, the Momentum Phase. This second phase of training, which will be followed for a total of four weeks (28 days), will turn the tables on prefatiguing the muscle. This time, strength and muscle development is the priority, which you will accomplish by completing a compound movement (focus on multiple muscles), then an isolation movement (focus on a single muscle). The goal of this phase is to reach failure at a lower rep range by using heavier weights to ensure that you build muscle onto the foundation you have spent five weeks creating. By performing exercises in this order—from compound to isolation—you will also add density to the muscle, which is a good thing since the denser the muscle, the more calories are burned to maintain it—this is when your body starts to turn into a calorie-burning machine.

You'll also increase the volume a bit in phase two, which means you will be completing four to five sets instead of just three. Increasing the number of sets will further boost calorie

TRANSFORMATION TRIGGERS—PHASE 2

MIND-SET MOTIVATION

If the mental stress of work is a burden, before you start your workout watch a motivational workout video on the Internet, stop at the coffee shop, or revisit chapters of this book—do whatever it takes to refocus your mind on *you* instead of your family/work environment. I personally drive home from the office and drink my coffee, take my pre-workout supplement, then watch a hard-core bodybuilding training DVD. Although the athletes' physiques aren't my ideal, the motivation, adrenaline, and intensity are things I want to emulate in order to transform my own physique in the gym. All of a sudden, I have forgotten about my deadlines, e-mails, and meetings and am now focused only on transforming my body.

PHYSICAL PREPARATION

As you begin to get stronger in the gym, your skeletal and tendon strength also becomes stronger, but at a much slower rate. For this reason, I recommend you purchase a weight belt to support your lower back on your heaviest back exercises and while performing squats. This will greatly support your back and assist with correct posture during training. Though this is recommended, it is not essential.

INSTANT INSPIRATION

"We are in control of our fitness. As long as we set our minds and determination towards fitness and do it despite any obstacles that we can use as an excuse, we give our bodies no choice but to become fit and healthy."

—Jeff *jeffasl*

burning, enhance muscle density, add strength, and give your muscles a rounder or fuller—not to be confused with bulkier—appearance.

You will notice too that I've given your cardio a boost in this phase. I've added just 5 minutes, so you're up to a total of 25 minutes. Your P.M. Cardio has also graduated to P.M. Cardio Plus, which means you're going to add in a quick abdominals session after your walk.

These two additions will stimulate faster metabolism of foods and take your fat loss up a notch.

When you make these strategic changes to your workouts starting in Week 6, you will be impressed by how they begin to accelerate your results. You should feel strong, confident, and driven—especially as the shape of your *real* body starts to show itself; get ready to start hearing compliments from the people around you right about now.

Take a look at the sample trackers for the Momentum Phase—you'll notice it's similar to the one from the first phase in terms of how to use it, so it should be pretty simple to make the switch to this new tracker.

> You should feel strong, confident, and driven—especially as the shape of your *real* body starts to show itself; get ready to start hearing compliments from the people around you.

THE BODY BY DESIGN PLAN

Phase 2, Day 1: Back and Biceps

DAY 1

Date: 2/14
Day __1__ of 28

A.M. Cardio (25 minutes) ☒

EXERCISE	SET 1: TR	WEIGHT/ AR	SET 2: TR	WEIGHT/ AR	SET 3: TR	WEIGHT/ AR	SET 4: TR	WEIGHT/ AR	SET 5: TR	WEIGHT/ AR
Lateral Pulldowns	10	60 lbs/ 10	10	60 lbs/ 10	10	60 lbs/ 10	10	60 lbs/ 10		
Reverse-grip Pulldowns	10	60 lbs/ 10	10	60 lbs/ 10	10	60 lbs/ 10	10	60 lbs/ 10		
Bent-over Dumbbell Rows	10	30 lbs/ 10	10	30 lbs/ 10	10	30 lbs/ 10	10	30 lbs/ 10		
Dumbbell Deadlifts	10	20 lbs/ 10	10	20 lbs/ 10	10	20 lbs/ 10	20	20 lbs/ 10		
Dumbbell Shrugs	10	40 lbs/ 10	10	40 lbs/ 10	10	40 lbs/ 10				
Barbell Curls	10	40 lbs/ 10	10	40 lbs/ 10	10	40 lbs/ 7	10	30 lbs/ 10	10	30 lbs/ 10
Preacher Curls	10	30 lbs/ 10	10	30 lbs/ 10	10	30 lbs/ 10	10	30 lbs/ 10	10	30 lbs/ 10

Phase 2, Day 2: Cardio, Upper Abdominals, and Cardio Plus

DAY 2

Date: 2/15
Day __2__ of 28

A.M. Cardio (25 minutes) ☒
P.M. Cardio (25 minutes) ☒

EXERCISE	SET 1: TR	AR	SET 2: TR	AR	SET 3: TR	AR	SET 4: TR	AR
A.M.: Abdominal Crunches	To failure	25	To failure	25	To failure	25		
P.M. PLUS: Twists	75/ side	75/side						

NOTES

Love this new phase—really feel like the extra sets created a new challenge. Push crunches up to at least 30 reps next time—you can do it! Fatigued on 3rd set of barbell curls—had to drop weight to 30 lbs on last two sets.

Phase 2, Day 3: Chest and Triceps

DAY 3

Date: 2/16
Day __3__ of 28

A.M. Cardio (25 minutes) ☒

EXERCISE	SET 1: TR	WEIGHT/ AR	SET 2: TR	WEIGHT/ AR	SET 3: TR	WEIGHT/ AR	SET 4: TR	WEIGHT/ AR	SET 5: TR	WEIGHT/ AR
Dumbbell Bench Press	10	45 lbs/ 10	10	45 lbs/ 10	10	45 lbs/ 10	10	45 lbs/ 10		
Straight-arm Dumbbell Pullovers	10	50 lbs/ 10	10	50 lbs/ 10	10	50 lbs/ 10	10	50 lbs/ 10		
Incline Dumbbell Press	10	45 lbs/ 10	10	45 lbs/ 10	10	45 lbs/ 30	10	45 lbs/ 10		
Incline Dumbbell Flyes	10	30 lbs/ 10	10	30 lbs/ 10	10	30 lbs/ 10	10	30 lbs/ 10		
Bench Dips	10	0/15	10	20 lbs/ 10	10	20 lbs/ 10	10	20 lbs/ 10		
Triceps Cable Extensions	10	70 lbs/ 10	10	70 lbs/ 10	10	70 lbs/ 10	10	70 lbs/ 10		
One-arm Triceps Dumbbell Extenions	10	25 lbs/ 10	10	25 lbs/ 10	10	25 lbs/ 10	10	25 lbs/ 10		

Phase 2, Day 4: Cardio, Upper Abdominals, and Cardio Plus

DAY 4

Date: 2/17
Day __4__ of 28

A.M. Cardio (25 minutes) ☒
P.M. Cardio (25 minutes) ☒

EXERCISE	SET 1: TR	AR	SET 2: TR	AR	SET 3: TR	AR	SET 4: TR	AR
A.M.: Lying Leg Raises	20	20	20	20	20	20		
P.M. PLUS: Twists	75/ side	75/side						

NOTES

Found bench dips easy—added 20 lb. barbell plate across my lap for more resistance.

Key: TR=Target Reps; AR=Actual Reps

Phase 2, Day 5: Shoulder and Legs

DAY 5

Date: 2/18
Day __5__ of 28

A.M. Cardio (25 minutes) ☒

EXERCISE	SET 1: TR	WEIGHT/ AR	SET 2: TR	WEIGHT/ AR	SET 3: TR	WEIGHT/ AR	SET 4: TR	WEIGHT/ AR	SET 5: TR	WEIGHT/ AR
Dumbbell Shoulder Press	10	40 lbs/ 10	10	40 lbs/ 10	10	40 lbs/ 10	10	40 lbs/ 10		
Bent-over Rear Raises	10	25 lbs/ 10	10	25 lbs/ 10	10	25 lbs/ 10	10	25 lbs/ 10		
Side Dumbbell Raises	10	25 lbs/ 10	10	25 lbs/ 10	10	25 lbs/ 10	10	25 lbs/ 10		
Front Dumbbell Raises	10	25 lbs/ 10	10	25 lbs/ 10	10	25 lbs/ 10	10	25 lbs/ 10		
Squats	20	70 lbs/ 20	20	70 lbs/ 20	20	70 lbs/ 20				
Leg Extensions	20	70 lbs/ 20	20	70 lbs/ 20	20	70 lbs/ 20				
Lying Leg Curls	15	60 lbs/ 15	15	60 lbs/ 15	15	60 lbs/ 15				
Leg Press	15	200 lbs/ 15	15	200 lbs/ 15	15	200 lbs/ 15				
Standing Calf Raises	10	100 lbs/ 10	10	100 lbs/ 10	10	100 lbs/ 10				
Seated Calf Raises	20	45 lbs/ 20	20	45 lbs/ 20	20	45 lbs/ 20				

Phase 2, Days 6: Cardio and Cardio Plus

DAY 6

Date: 2/19
Day __6__ of 28

A.M. Cardio (25 minutes) ☒
P.M. Cardio (25 minutes) ☒

EXERCISE	SET 1: TR	AR	SET 2: TR	AR	SET 3: TR	AR	SET 4: TR	AR
P.M. PLUS: Twists	75/ side	75/side						

Phase 2, Days 7: Cardio and Cardio Plus

DAY 7

Date: 2/20
Day __7__ of 28

A.M. Cardio (25 minutes) ☒
P.M. Cardio (25 minutes) ☒

EXERCISE	SET 1: TR	AR	SET 2: TR	AR	SET 3: TR	AR	SET 4: TR	AR
P.M. PLUS: Twists	75/ side	75/side						

NOTES

3. THE DTP PHASE (WEEKS 10–12)

The final stage of the Body by Design workout plan incorporates a training principle I've refined over the years through my work with clients and in my own workouts. This phase will turn your already great results into outstanding ones. By following only the first two phases of the program, I'm certain you will have produced incredible results, and you may have even reached your goal already. If you haven't and you really want to push your body to the next level, performing exercises using the Dramatic Transformation Principle (DTP) will create the challenge you need to reveal sensational results. At this stage, I consider you to be of advanced level and physically and mentally prepared for the three-week (21-day) DTP Phase.

The exercises in phase three are very simple, so I don't want you to feel intimidated when I use the word "advanced"; I simply mean that you have put in the work to prepare your body for this phase; you are ready for it, and I wouldn't be including it here if you weren't. You'll notice that the exercises are similar to those in the Momentum Phase; however, the way they are performed is very different. By introducing the DTP, you'll place a new and distinct stress on your muscles and push your body to produce previously unimaginable results—yes, you're going to want to break out the sleeveless shirts and backless dresses. The physical results develop so fast in this phase

(as long as you're following the cardio and nutrition elements) that I recommend you follow it for no more than three weeks. Failure to limit this intense training phase will lead to overtraining and compromise your long-term results.

HOW IT WORKS

In the DTP Phase, each workout includes two paired exercises that have been strategically selected to focus on specific muscle groups. The pairings are designed to mostly train antagonistic (opposing) muscle groups. On day one, I've paired the chest and back muscle groups, and on day three, the biceps and triceps. The last combination, which you will complete on day five, is slightly different because it puts two compound exercises back to back—one for legs (squats) and one for shoulders (dumbbell shoulder press). With these strategic pairings, the muscle fibers are totally broken down while the opposing muscle is recovering and no other exercise is needed for either muscle group. You'll be performing these exercises in supersets, which means that instead of completing all your sets for one exercise like you've done before, you will complete two exercises back to back with no rest (you will rest for 45 seconds after you complete a set of each, or one superset).

The first warm-up set is counted as a working set due to the high number of reps performed. During the first six sets, the goal is to increase (pyramid) the weight on every set.

You will begin the first set with a light weight and perform 50 reps; then you will add weight and decrease the number of reps until you get to 5; it will look like this: 50 reps, 40 reps, 30 reps, 20 reps, 10 reps, 5 reps. Then you need to mirror this rep structure for the remaining six sets, but you will *decrease* the weight on each set as you work your way back up to 50 reps. Your sets will look like this: 5 reps, 10 reps, 20 reps, 30 reps, 40 reps, 50 reps. Before you get confused, let me guide you through an example.

Using two exercises, barbell curls and lying triceps extensions, I'm going to describe how I would perform these exercises with the DTP so you get see a very clear picture. I begin by selecting a light weight for my barbell curls and perform 50 reps; hopefully, I've selected the right weight so I will reach failure at the right point (of course, I'll keep track of the weight

TRANSFORMATION TRIGGERS—PHASE 3

MIND-SET MOTIVATION

As you start to push your body further, I want you to add a visualization technique for optimizing performance during your workouts. Just before you perform a set, close your eyes and visualize yourself wearing the same clothes you are at that moment, performing the number of reps required. Imagine how the muscles contract and stretch during this exercise, feel how the weight sits in your hands, breathe at the rate you would. When it's time to begin the set in real time, you have already completed it; you just have to go through the movements. A lot of professional athletes I've trained use this visualization technique before training or before big fights or games—it's a powerful method for achieving your best, no matter what the activity.

PHYSICAL PREPARATION

During the DTP phase you may notice hunger cravings even though you're eating six meals per day. You are really pushing your body to produce phenomenal results at this point; any little bit of extra hunger you feel is your body burning through fat for energy; it's taking those final steps before the big unveil of the lean, toned muscle you've been building over the past nine weeks. To help combat any cravings, even though it may sound obvious, be sure you're eating all your meals—if you're not paying attention, it's easy to accidentally skip a meal. (Read about what to eat in the next chapter.) I also encourage you to make extra efforts to take special care of your body during this phase: get plenty of sleep so you can recover energy and replenish the hormones that help balance stress and hunger; drink plenty of water, which will keep your energy levels up and make sure you don't mistake thirst for hunger.

BODY BY DESIGN SAMPLE DTP PHASE WORKOUT TRACKER

Phase 3, Day 1: Chest and Back

DAY 1

Date: 3/14
Day __1__ of 21

A.M. Cardio (30 minutes) ☒

	EXERCISE 1	EXERCISE 2		EXERCISE 1	EXERCISE 2
	Dumbbell Bench Press	Bent-over Dumbbell Rows		Dumbbell Bench Press	Bent-over Dumbbell Rows
Set 1: TR	50	50	Set 7: TR	5	5
Weight/AR	30 lbs/50	20 lbs/50	Weight/AR	70 lbs/5	60 lbs/5
Set 2: TR	40	40	Set 8: TR	10	10
Weight/AR	40 lbs/40	30 lbs/40	Weight/AR	60 lbs/10	50 lbs/10
Set 3: TR	30	30	Set 9: TR	20	20
Weight/AR	50 lbs/30	40 lbs/30	Weight/AR	50 lbs/20	40 lbs/20
Set 4: TR	20	20	Set 10: TR	30	30
Weight/AR	60 lbs/20	50 lbs/20	Weight/AR	40 lbs/30	30 lbs/30
Set 5: TR	10	10	Set 11: TR	40	40
Weight/AR	70 lbs/10	60 lbs/10	Weight/AR	30 lbs/40	20 lbs/40
Set 6: TR	5	5	Set 12: TR	50	50
Weight/AR	80 lbs/5	70 lbs/5	Weight/AR	15 lbs/50	20 lbs/50

Phase 3, Day 2: Cardio, Upper and Lower Abdominals, and Cardio Plus

DAY 2

Date: 3/15
Day __2__ of 21

A.M. Cardio (30 minutes) ☒
P.M. Cardio (30 minutes) ☒

EXERCISE	SET 1: TR	AR	SET 2: TR	AR	SET 3: TR	AR	SET 4: TR	AR
A.M.: Lying Leg Raises	25	25	25	25	25	25		
A.M.: Abdominal Crunches	25	25	25	25	25	25		
P.M. PLUS: Twists	75/side	75/side						

NOTES

Can't believe I'm already at the DTP phase! A tough workout, but I was ready for it. Don't rush through sets next time & be sure to maintain form.

Phase 3, Day 3: Biceps and Triceps

DAY 3

Date: 3/16
Day __3__ of 21

A.M. Cardio (30 minutes) ☒

	EXERCISE 1	EXERCISE 2		EXERCISE 1	EXERCISE 2
	Barbell Curls	**Lying Triceps Extensions**		**Barbell Curls**	**Lying Triceps Extensions**
Set 1: TR	50	50	Set 7: TR	5	5
Weight/AR	20 lbs/50	25 lbs/50	Weight/AR	55 lbs/5	65 lbs/5
Set 2: TR	40	40	Set 8: TR	10	10
Weight/AR	25 lbs/40	30 lbs/40	Weight/AR	45 lbs/10	55 lbs/10
Set 3: TR	30	30	Set 9: TR	20	20
Weight/AR	30 lbs/30	35 lbs/30	Weight/AR	35 lbs/20	45 lbs/20
Set 4: TR	20	20	Set 10: TR	30	30
Weight/AR	35 lbs/20	45 lbs/20	Weight/AR	30 lbs/30	35 lbs/30
Set 5: TR	10	10	Set 11: TR	40	40
Weight/AR	45 lbs/10	55 lbs/10	Weight/AR	25 lbs/40	30 lbs/40
Set 6: TR	5	5	Set 12: TR	50	50
Weight/AR	55 lbs/5	65 lbs/5	Weight/AR	20 lbs/50	25 lbs/50

Phase 3, Day 4: Cardio, Upper and Lower Abdominals, and Cardio Plus

DAY 4

Date: 3/17
Day __4__ of 21

A.M. Cardio (30 minutes) ☒
P.M. Cardio (30 minutes) ☒

EXERCISE	SET 1: TR	AR	SET 2: TR	AR	SET 3: TR	AR	SET 4: TR	AR
A.M.: Abdominal Crunches	25	25	25	25	25	25		
A.M.: Lying Leg Raises	25	25	25	25	25	25		
P.M. PLUS: Twists	75/side	75/side						

NOTES

108

Phase 3, Day 5: Legs and Shoulders

DAY 5

Date: 3/18
Day __5__ of 21

A.M. Cardio (30 minutes) ☒

	EXERCISE 1	EXERCISE 2		EXERCISE 1	EXERCISE 2
	Squats	Dumbbell Shoulder Press		Squats	Dumbbell Shoulder Press
Set 1: TR	50	50	Set 7: TR	5	5
Weight/AR	0/50	15 lbs/50	Weight/AR	80 lbs/5	50 lbs/5
Set 2: TR	40	40	Set 8: TR	10	10
Weight/AR	10 lbs/40	20 lbs/40	Weight/AR	55 lbs/10	35 lbs/10
Set 3: TR	30	30	Set 9: TR	20	20
Weight/AR	20 lbs/30	25 lbs/30	Weight/AR	35 lbs/20	30 lbs/20
Set 4: TR	20	20	Set 10: TR	30	30
Weight/AR	35 lbs/20	30 lbs/20	Weight/AR	20 lbs/30	25 lbs/30
Set 5: TR	10	10	Set 11: TR	40	40
Weight/AR	55 lbs/10	35 lbs/10	Weight/AR	10 lbs/40	20 lbs/40
Set 6: TR	5	5	Set 12: TR	50	50
Weight/AR	80 lbs/5	50 lbs/5	Weight/AR	0/50	15 lbs/50

Phase 3, Day 6: Cardio and Cardio Plus

DAY 6

Date: 3/19
Day __6__ of 21

A.M. Cardio (30 minutes) ☒
P.M. Cardio (30 minutes) ☒

EXERCISE	SET 1: TR	AR	SET 2: TR	AR	SET 3: TR	AR	SET 4: TR	AR
P.M. PLUS: Twists	75/side	75/side						

Phase 3, Day 7: Cardio and Cardio Plus

DAY 7

Date: 3/20
Day __7__ of 21

A.M. Cardio (30 minutes) ☒
P.M. Cardio (30 minutes) ☒

EXERCISE	SET 1: TR	AR	SET 2: TR	AR	SET 3: TR	AR	SET 4: TR	AR
P.M. PLUS: Twists	75/side	75/side						

NOTES

As I lowered my reps while doing squats, I noticed a large increase in strength so my weight used jumped significantly the last couple of sets.

Key: TR=Target Reps; AR=Actual Reps

used and make any notes about increasing or decreasing the weight on my workout tracker so I can refer back to it next time). I immediately follow that exercise with 50 reps of lying triceps extensions. I'm starting to feel nice and warmed up, but I take a quick 45-second rest to let my breath recover. Then I choose a weight that will allow me to reach failure on both exercises at 40 reps, followed again by a 45-second rest. I continue in the same pattern over the next four sets until failure is reached at 5 reps. Once I've finished going up the pyramid in weight and down it in reps, it's time to reverse the pattern: I'm now going to work from my heaviest weight down to my lowest and from the lowest number of reps to the highest, eventually ending up back at 50 reps. Let me use the workout tracker to demonstrate this visually, since I've increased the number of sets and decreased the number of exercises performed, you will notice this tracker looks different from those we used in the first two phases.

Don't be intimidated by the number of sets you see in the DTP Phase Workout Tracker; focus instead on the fact that you are performing only two exercises on each workout day. The key is to maintain proper form and breathing through every rep you complete; since you are completing a high number of reps, a lack of concentration on each and every one could lead to poor form, which inevitably leads to compromised results or even injury. Remember, your total workout should be less than an

INSTANT INSPIRATION

"If I could give one piece of advice it would be to stay *consistent* <http://www
.bodybuilding.com/fun/bbinfo.php?page=Dedication> and be patient. The weight
didn't come on overnight, and it will not go away overnight. Surround yourself
with like-minded positive people and know that you don't have to be a movie star
to have the body you want. All you need is a made up mind."

—Christi*BabyBeFit38

hour, so stay true to the commitments you've made to yourself by making every minute count.

Now that you have a complete understanding of the Body by Design workout program, let's talk about what can make or break the ultimate outcome of your transformation: the eating plan. I strongly recommend you read Chapter 8, "The Body by Design Eating Plan," before starting your workouts, but as soon as you're ready to hit the weights, remember to go to the Exercise Database on page 147 for exercise descriptions and images.

"It's like I've Been REBORN."

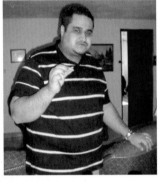

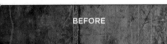

BEFORE

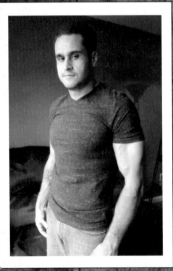

AFTER

"I tried to lose weight countless times and failed," says Claudio Ramos. "Sometimes you have to fail at something many times to finally succeed once. I had accepted being big and had adjusted myself to the lifestyle. I would eat junk food and drink sodas all day—nutrition didn't matter to me. I drank alcohol on the weekends and never exercised. All of these things combined led to my health issues."

At 25, he was 317 pounds, borderline diabetic, and suffering from severe sleep apnea. "I was just in bad shape altogether," recalls Claudio, who adds that the physical struggles were only part of the problem. "Getting over the mental state of mind—the thought that I would never be able to lose weight—was the toughest obstacle," he says.

He started his transformation with walking and started to see results. "This gave me the motivation to continue," he says. "So I started to eat healthy, which led to more weight loss. Then I added weight training, which really started to create change in my body." Claudio went on to lose an incredible 135 pounds, going from 317 to a muscular and fit 182. "I truly never thought I would lose this amount of weight."

His transformation was so profound that he feels as though he's living a brand-new life. "It's like I've been reborn," he says. "I have changed so much that I almost forgot what my life was like before—this is literally a new lease on life."

Claudio credits BodySpace for playing a significant role in his transformation, particularly the connections and the system of accountability he found there. "It helped me tremendously," he says. "The site gave me the chance to connect with people who share the same goals as I do and exchange successes and struggles with them—we are there to help each other. The motivation and dedication from the people I've connected with on BodySpace gave me the strength to continue and push harder. They also keep me going at all times because it's like a promise I've made—I can't quit because they're watching my success and waiting to encourage me, and I'm doing the same for them."

Another reason for his success is that he finally stopped trying fad diets and instead created a new lifestyle for himself. "Fad diets seem to work initially, but then they fail miserably," he says.

"I finally learned how to train, what to eat, and when to eat it. I discovered that there is no magic pill or fad diet that works—it truly has to become part of your lifestyle."

Making it a lifestyle included ensuring that his kitchen wasn't filled with things that would detract from his commitments to health. "All the junk food was removed from my house and replaced with good, nutritious foods," he says, and acknowledges that he couldn't have created a healthy home without the support of his wife, Melissa. "I also stopped drinking altogether, cut out sodas and juices, and drank only water. I really believe that seventy-five percent of success comes from nutrition."

He now finds himself energized and ready to face every day. "Sleep apnea used to take a great amount of energy away from me, and since losing weight I don't have that anymore," he notes. He also takes pride in his new physical abilities. "I can actually run now, and I can finally pick up my own weight and do pull-ups and chin-ups. I can't remember the last time I felt so good and healthy."

Renewed confidence about his body and looks has helped improve his life in ways he never would have expected. "Before I always had this self-conscious, nervous feeling like I was the center of attention," he says, "but in a bad way because of the way I looked; I would get anxiety and start sweating for no reason." Since his transformation, those feelings have disappeared. "It feels like a load has been lifted. I am very confident about the way I look now, and I feel great. My transformation was for health reasons, but I never knew I would experience a therapeutic kind of pride about who I've become."

With confidence and a whole new outlook on life, Claudio now finds himself looking forward to the future—and even planning for it. "Before my transformation, I had no goals," he says. "I had no ambition because I thought my time had come and gone. Now I want to reach for the sky."

> "I can't remember the last time I felt so good and healthy."

From Losing Everything to a RENEWED
Sense of PURPOSE

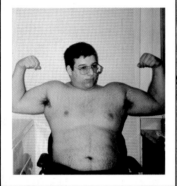

BEFORE

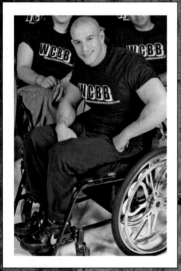

AFTER

When Nick Scott was told he was never going to be able to walk again, he remembers feeling as though a part of him had died. "At the same time, another part was born," he says. "I realized the one thing you gain from losing everything is perspective. At that point it wasn't about whether the glass was half empty or half full; I was just grateful to have a glass."

Nick was still in high school when the accident that changed his life happened; thinking back, he can remember the moment he chose which path to take. "I was in rehab in Topeka for four weeks," he recalls. "For once since the accident, I was alone, and it hit me that I hadn't seen what I looked like, so I found a mirror. My weight had gone up to about 300 pounds; I had grown a mini-Afro and a spotted beard and just felt like a freak," he says. "And at that point I told myself I would never look like that again."

He knew he would have to get back into the gym to rebuild strength and lose weight, but he faced the challenge of working out with a completely different body. "I thought going back to weight lifting would make me feel better; I was wrong, and it was the total opposite," he says. "It killed me to see everybody do the things that I couldn't do." He felt at a loss, but not for long. "Then finally it dawned on me—I decided if I couldn't do anything, the one thing I could be is stronger than everybody. I started bench-pressing again and had someone help me lie down on the bench, stand on my feet, and hold my knees. That was the turning point."

At first, everything was a challenge. "In the gym I didn't feel stable with a lot of things, and trying to lift made me feel more unstable with certain exercises," he remembers. "It was constantly a struggle in the beginning, but if I wanted to change I had no choice except to figure it out—and that's what I did. I just kept with it and learned as time went on. Eventually everything became easier because my core became stronger, my balance got better, and transforming was so much easier."

Even though his disability has provided tougher obstacles than some face, Nick feels that his transformational process is something everyone can relate to. "We all have problems in our lives and we all have challenges and we all have disabilities," he says, "it's just that mine is physical. For all of us, it's about pushing ourselves to overcome that obstacle or task that faces us. If we can learn to just not give up and just think that there is a way, then we will succeed at anything we do."

When he felt that he had reached a confident level of fitness, Nick decided to look into wheelchair bodybuilding, hoping that competing would help him take it up a notch. After participating in a competition (he came in second—even though he would have preferred first), he returned home with a renewed interest in the sport. "I discovered there was barely anything online about it, and I decided I wanted the world to know about the sport," he says. So he went to work creating a Web site. "I taught myself how to build a Web site and did a lot of research and made a simple site so anybody can find what they're looking for quickly. It took off, and wheelchair bodybuilders around the world contact me all the time wanting to compete or get in shape."

He encourages others to focus on establishing precise goals when it comes to creating change. "With clear and defined goals, you can focus and know exactly what you are trying to achieve." He also stresses the importance of eating right. "Many people overlook the significance of nutrition," he notes. "People will spend many hours working out but never understand why they don't look good in the mirror. There are 168 hours in a week, and only a small number of them are spent in the gym."

With a commitment to fitness, Nick has changed his life. "For me, fitness is not just going to the gym to workout; it is a lifestyle," he says. "I have become stronger from within and have seen and done things I never thought possible. I am grateful for all the doors that were put before me and that I found something deep inside to push me through them."

"With clear and defined goals, you can focus and know exactly what you are trying to achieve."

CHAPTER 8

The Body by Design

EATING
PLAN

As in the good old debate about the chicken and egg, you might wonder what comes first when you really get down to changing your body: diet or exercise? Though you certainly can't truly transform your body without exercise, specifically strength training, the quality and quantity of food you put into your body nudge out exercise by a nose when it comes to laying the groundwork for your transformation. The food you eat provides your body with the nutrients and materials it needs to construct cells an important tissues, such as muscle. It also contributes to the energy exchange, known as your metabolism, that keeps your body running; food provides the units of energy (calories) that your body burns through or stores as fat for future use. Though it's a bit more complex than simply "calories in, calories out," the basic point of that phrase is true: what you put in is put back out in the form of energy—or, if you've consumed more calories than you need, you gain weight.

For this reason, your diet is key to creating change in your body; in fact, you could lose weight by just consuming a low-calorie diet. What you can't do is create fat-burning muscle and a strong and toned shape that will rejuvenate and transform your life. People who lose weight with diet alone develop a flat, shapeless appearance, not a fit, lively, head-turning one.

WHAT TO EAT

Now let's take a look at the specifics of the Body by Design eating plan. I've kept it as simple as possible so you can quickly and easily apply it to your life.

1. You need to eat every two to three hours, or about six times per day
2. You should eat more whole foods–based meals but supplement with meal replacement shakes when needed
3. Every meal should consist of:

➤ A palm-sized protein source with a palm-sized carbohydrate source

➤ A fist-sized portion of vegetables
➤ One tablespoon of a condiment

4. And, to ensure optimum success, you should:

➤ Drink one gallon of water a day
➤ Add supplements that will help boost your performance and muscle recovery

That's the eating plan boiled down to just a few core points; you are welcome to hit the ground running with just that powerful bit of information, but I suggest you read on so you're fully armed with all the tools and knowledge you need. I've broken down the plan into three core categories: Frequency, Foods, and Supplements.

FREQUENCY

If you are motivated and ready for a successful transformation, you have to answer "yes" to the following question:

Can you eat every three hours?

Eating at frequent intervals is imperative if you want your body to be a fat-burning furnace. When you eat every three hours, about six meals a day, it's just like feeding a flame with high-quality fuel—the more you feed it, the stronger the fat-burning flame will be. Fueling your body frequently will keep your blood sugar level stable, reducing cravings; feed your muscles, giving them power and strength; and provide your brain and body with functional energy.

If you find it physically hard to eat a solid meal six times per day (most of us do), you can have a protein or meal replacement shake as a substitute. However, I don't want you to abuse the privilege of having a protein shake whenever you feel like it to satisfy convenience and your taste buds. I prefer to have my shakes only after workouts or when I'm really craving something sweet—a chocolate protein shake can be your best ally when it comes to defeating cravings. Aim to have no more than three shakes per day (including your postworkout shake), and don't have two shakes in a row. The reason for this is that whole foods are more thermogenic and require more calories to digest, so they are superior to supplement-based shakes. Most shakes are very high in their bioavailability, which means they absorb quickly and effectively, but the body requires the sustenance that it has been accustomed to for thousands of years: real food.

FOODS

What you'll be eating on this plan can be broken down into four categories: protein, carbohydrates, vegetables, and condiments. Remember, the portions per meal are palm-sized for protein, palm-sized for carbohydrate, fist-sized for vegetables, and a tablespoon of condiment. These are the portions recommended for most of your six meals through-

out the day. On average, this will amount to about a 6-to-8-ounce serving of protein or six egg whites; 3/4 cup of your carbohydrate source, cooked; and 1 cup of vegetables, raw or cooked. The portion size will vary based on the size of your hands, which is why it's the perfect measurement and the simplest way to customize how much food (and how many calories) you eat. Don't be too concerned about your portions of vegetables or salad—they contain plenty of water, are a good source of fiber, and have very few calories, so you can't really eat too much. Here's a general guideline for your food portions (the condiment portion of one tablespoon is the same for everyone, regardless of body size):

Food Type	Customized Measurement	Average Portion Size
Protein	Palm-sized	6 ounces
Carbohydrate	Palm-sized	Approximately 3/4 cup
Vegetable	Fist-sized	Approximately 1 cup

INSTANT INSPIRATION

"You are powerful, sensitive, determined, and gracious—I can see you achieving everything you choose to achieve. I can see you being exactly who and what you want to be. You can accomplish anything—I know you can. Eat right, stay around positive people, and make every day the best day of your life."

—Jessica*Dr.Euphoria

On page 120, you will find an Approved Foods table that tells you precisely what foods to eat on this plan. The only fats I recommend during your twelve-week transformation are those that naturally occur in your protein sources, such as steak, chicken, and fish, so you won't see a separate category for fats. If you have an unbearable craving every now and again, you can have some celery topped with about a tablespoon of natural peanut butter—this is the perfect amount of satisfying, healthy fat that will help you overcome that craving.

There are a couple of rules you can stretch within this program, although that doesn't mean you can *break* the rules entirely. For example, it can be tough to get protein, carbs, *and* vegetables at each meal. Let's say you mix protein powder in with some oatmeal for breakfast, which would fulfill your protein and carbs—are you going to want to add some salsa and broccoli? I don't think so. That's okay. The main sources of foods I want you to concentrate on for the first four meals of the day (until about 3 P.M.) are protein and carbohydrates.

After 3 P.M., I want you to cut out the starchier types of carbohydrates, such as potatoes and pasta, and enjoy your last two meals with vegetables. Vegetables are an incredible source of vital nutrients, and they have very few calories compared to more complex carbohydrates such as brown rice and potatoes. For the last two meals at night, you don't need these extra calories since you've more than likely fueled your day already. When sleeping, you won't have a chance to burn off any complex carbohydrates, which is why we cut them from the last hours of the day. Here's an example of a pre–3 P.M. meal and a post–3 P.M. meal:

➤ **Pre–3 P.M.:** A palm-sized amount of grilled chicken breast, chopped, and a palm-sized serving of boiled or steamed brown rice, served with a fist-sized amount of mushrooms, lettuce, and cucumber, topped with a tablespoon of salsa.

➤ **Post–3 P.M.:** A palm-sized serving of grilled lean steak with broccoli, mushrooms, and peppers, sautéed with a tablespoon of soy sauce.

Please remember one of the most important factors of the nutrient plan: if it isn't included in the Approved Foods table on page 120, assume you cannot eat it. Deli meat isn't included, so assume you cannot eat it; the same goes for fruit, milk, breakfast bars, cereals, nuts, and so on. Sticking to the foods you see in the table will ensure that you achieve a jaw-dropping transformation in just twelve weeks.

The distinguishing factor between healthful eating and transformational eating is the calorie content and the form the calories come in. Fruit contains a sugar (fructose), which is much better than table sugar (sucrose), but it is still a fast-burning carb that needs to be burned off. Milk and most dairy products contain another sugar (lactose), which is another calorie source you don't want to be burning off while

BODY BY DESIGN APPROVED FOODS			
PROTEIN	**CARBOHYDRATES**	**VEGGIES/SALAD/FRUIT**	**CONDIMENTS**
Chicken breast	Brown rice	Broccoli	Fat-free Italian dressing
Lean steak	Wholemeal pancakes	Mushroom	Fat-free French dressing
Turkey breast	Whole wheat pasta	Tomato	Mustards (easy on the whole grains)
Egg whites	Sweet potato	Lettuce	Salsa
Protein powder	Yam	Cabbage	Balsamic vinegar
Veal	Potato	Cucumber	Lemon or lime juice
Fat-free cottage cheese	Rolled oats or oatmeal	Cauliflower	Pickle relish
Soy	GENr8 Vitargo	Spinach	Soy sauce
Whitefish	Whole wheat bread	Celery	Fresh herbs and garlic Chili powder (no oil)
Salmon	Whole wheat tortilla	Zucchini	Cooking spray

you are on the treadmill—you should instead be burning off body fat. If you can't imagine your life without fruit or dairy products for twelve weeks, you can try a few of my emergency exceptions: for dairy, try a serving of high-quality Greek yogurt, such as FAGE, or fat-free cheese; for fruit, an apple or a few chunks of pineapple. To produce maximum results, I recommend avoiding these foods or using them to fulfill only the most intense of cravings.

Please check out the Approved Foods table and get to know the foods that are going to help you build and sculpt your brand-new body.

I believe in a straightforward, simple approach to nutrition, which is why I've left out overly scientific nutritional information that you don't need to know for your transformation (if you want to become a true student of nutrition, you can check out some of the free content at www.bodybuilding.com). To help you get started, I've included a sample nutrition tracker for your first day. Since day one will be a workout day, it's important that you consume the proper post workout meal. The combination of protein powder, Vitargo, and creatine ("meal 5") is ideal for replenishing muscles. I recommend only consuming Vitargo and creatine on training days as part of your post workout meal—on off days, your body won't be in need of their fast-acting qualities.

Date: 1/10

Day _____ of 84

Water (1 gallon) ☒

MEAL 1

Protein: 2 scoops protein powder

Carbs: 3/4 cup rolled oats

Veggies: ————

Condiments: ————

Time: 6:30 A.M.

MEAL 2

Protein: Palm-sized serving grilled chicken breast

Carbs: 3/4 cup cooked sweet potato

Veggies: Salad w/lettuce, alfalfa sprouts, & cucumber

Condiments: 1 tablespoon fat-free Italian dressing

Time: 9:30 A.M.

MEAL 3

Protein:

Carbs: ⟩ Chocolate MRP Shake

Veggies:

Condiments:

Time: NOON

MEAL 4

Protein: Omelet w/6 egg whites

Carbs: 3/4 cooked brown rice

Veggies: Bell peppers, tomatoes, & mushrooms (in omelet)

Condiments: 1 tablespoon salsa

Time: 3:00 P.M.

MEAL 5

Protein: 2 scoops protein powder

Veggies: ————   1-2 scoops vitargo (post workout)

Condiments: ————   1 serving creatine

Time: 6:00 P.M.

MEAL 6

Protein: Palm-sized fillet grilled salmon

Veggies: Steamed broccoli & cauliflower

Condiments: 1 tablespoon soy sauce

Time: 8:00 P.M.

Supplements:

Added BCAAs to water — loved the grape flavor. Took multivitamin morning & night.

Notes:

I wasn't hungry at all like I thought I would be — feeling full and healthy. Leave some hot sauce

at work to spice up chicken a bit. No veggies or condiments in meal 5—post-workout supplements gave me a great recharge.

This nutrition tracker example is for a workout day, so meal 5 happens to be supplement-based. This example can include more solid meals if desired. I personally have a shake only postworkout and when I have cravings. Other than that I prefer solid food choices because they are more satisfying and filling. Since the MRP shakes contain carbohydrates and a spectrum of vitamins and minerals, you should have them only during your first four meals; you can have protein shakes throughout the entire day.

One of the great things I find when I'm going through a personal transformation is the creative inspiration it gives me in the kitchen. You can also see my "spice it up" ideas in the table below—fresh ingredients, sauces, and spices that add substantial flavor without the extra fat or calories. If you are the kind of person who gets bored with food quickly, please

BODY BY DESIGN SPICE IT UP		
FRESH	SAUCE	SPICE
Ginger	Tapatío hot sauce	Cayenne pepper
Garlic	Tabasco	Black pepper
Cilantro	Cholula	Lemon pepper
Red or green onion	Siracha	Curry powder
Jalapeño	Frank's Red Hot Original Hot Sauce	Garlic powder
Lemon or lime juice	Soy sauce	Chili powder

check out the recipes in the Resources section. I have tried and tested every one of the recipes included there. You can also join the Body by Design BodyGroup online and exchange recipes and ideas with others who are following the plan. Visit www.bodybuilding.com/bodybydesign to find out more.

SUPPLEMENTS

Though supplements aren't a magic pill, they can add a significant element of convenience to your eating plan, which by now you know requires you to eat at frequent intervals. They can also provide a great sanctuary when cravings rear their ugly, uninvited heads. A favorite nighttime treat of mine is to mix a thick, creamy protein pudding powder and enjoy it with a stalk of celery. Okay, it's not exactly decadent—but it sure beats consuming a high-calorie cookie that would destroy all chances of a successful transformation.

As the editor in chief of Bodybuilding.com, I am in the unique position to know my way around a supplement shelf, and I have tried and tested almost everything I can pronounce. With so many supplements available, I take only the very basic ones. When I present them to you here, the list may seem long, but that is because most of the time I prefer to purchase single ingredients instead of blends; that way I know exactly what specific supplement, and how much of it, works best for me.

Next is the list of supplements that I take and also the ones I recommend to everyone

INSTANT INSPIRATION

"Each workout and each meal has a purpose—to help me achieve my goals. Working out and eating healthy has become a lifestyle, not just an activity I have to get motivated to do. I set goals and focus on achieving them."

—Jay*JAYcavalier_328

else seeking a top-notch transformation. I've spent more than a decade taking and refining my supplement list, and I have found this formula best fuels my workouts, helps me recover quickly, and also happens to satisfy my taste buds. These recommendations come from my own personal experience, and I'm not paid to push a specific brand or product.

1. A MULTIVITAMIN AND MULTIMINERAL FORMULA. Soil today is much more cultivated than it was in years past, which has greatly depleted the minerals and vitamins you get from the foods that grow in the soil and the animals that live off the land. This is why I highly recommend taking a multivitamin and multimineral formula morning and night to be sure your body is provided with all the nutrients it needs for good health that you may not be getting from the foods on your eating plan. I personally take the Gaspari Nutrition multivitamin called Anavite because it is designed to enhance performance for the active individual.

2. A PROTEIN POWDER. Try your best to eat a palm-sized portion of protein with every meal, as this will help your muscles rebuild and recover from the stress placed on them during workouts. Since eating protein six times per day can get a little inconvenient, you can try drinking it occasionally. If I know I'm going to have a lot of meetings in a day, I always pack my cooler bag, but sometimes I have to eat during meetings, which is tough and especially difficult if I have to do most of the talking. That's when I'll grab my shaker bottle that I've already scooped protein powder into, add a little water, and drink. Sometimes there's just no other option, and these quick, nutrient-rich shakes can be a lifesaver!

There are many great-tasting protein powders available, but I like the Gaspari Probiotic Myofusion because it is very low in lactose, tastes great, and contains good bacteria and probiotics, including acidophilus and bifidus. This shake can also be mixed thick in case I prefer a dessertlike consistency. I recommend you consume your protein shake as a meal replacement when carbohydrates aren't required and as your post-workout shake, mixed with carbohydrate powder and creatine (more on those supplements later). These shakes should be mixed with water, not milk, to avoid additional sugar.

3. A CARBOHYDRATE POWDER. Recent years have brought us a sense of paranoia about carbs; I truly don't understand the fuss. I love carbs, but I am educated enough to know which ones to eat and when. There are some that are digested very fast, such as those derived from white flour, and I do recommend you avoid these. However, there is a time and a place for fast-digesting carbs.

The good news is that there's a way to get those kinds of carbs without eating foods filled with sugar or white flour. The fastest of all is a powder called GENr8 Vitargo, which is a starch that contains no sugar but is digested by the body faster than a sugar. When your energy levels are at their most depleted, which is normally after a workout, it is essential to feed your body as soon as possible to ensure adequate restoration. That way, your muscles can perform at their best the following day and in later workouts. I personally have my protein shake with natural-flavored GENr8 Vitargo immediately postworkout, and I recommend you do the same. If you've trained hard, the carbohydrates will replenish your depleted energy stores and will not promote fat gain.

4. **BRANCHED-CHAIN AMINO ACIDS (BCAAS).** Branched-chain amino acids are three of the essential amino acids that make up the skeletal muscle in our bodies. Amino acids are the building blocks of protein, which your body uses to create muscle and other tissues. Because your body cannot produce these essential amino acids on its own—meaning it gets them from your diet—supplementing what you get from solid foods can help improve recovery, prevent muscle wastage, and promote protein synthesis. If you don't supply your body with enough BCAAs, it will break down muscle and tissues to use for energy—something you definitely want to avoid.

While that's a significant part of the reason I take BCAAs, another reason is that it makes me drink more water. I recommend the Xtend powder formula made by Scivation because it tastes great when you add it to water. I add several scoops to my gallon jug of water, and the water's gone before I know it. The grape flavor prompts me to drink much more water throughout the day than I would if it were tasteless. Plus, I think the little bit of sweetness helps ward off cravings. The Xtend brand also contains glutamine, which further enhances recovery and promotes a healthy immune system.

5. **FAT BURNERS.** This is a controversial topic, as there is no such thing as a "magic pill" that is going to help you lose those unwanted pounds. A good fat burner, however, can really help with all the aspects of a transformation that people tend to struggle with. The best I have found is called Grenade Thermo Detonator® ("Grenade Fat Burner"). The purpose of a fat burner is to help suppress appetite and control cravings, bolster mental focus, and perhaps most important increase energy to get the most out of each training session while on a diet of low carbs/calories. Grenade ticks

INSTANT INSPIRATION

"Just like piloting a plane, I want all the instrument needles of my life pointing in the right direction. Then I want to go to full power and climb to higher altitudes. I am motivated by the great people on BodySpace—their dedication, hard work, and the encouragement they provide."

—Chuck*ChuckFit40s

all of these boxes without any jitters, anxiety, or crash that I have experienced with similar products in the past. I take 1 capsule before my cardio sessions.

6. MEAL REPLACEMENT. Nutrition by Design Meals aren't considered supplements so much as real meals; however, they do have the convenience of supplements. These lean protein and slow release carbohydrate meals are perfect to eat on the go; all you need is boiling water and 8 minutes to allow it to cook. I like to take them with me while traveling, sitting at the office, driving in the car, or when I don't have time to grocery shop and prepare and cook a meal. They taste good in addition to being very satisfying. The chicken breast and lean beef options are perfectly balanced for those aiming to build muscle and burn fat for a successful transformation. These meals have been created under my own strict guidance so they can be conveniently enjoyed specifically as part of this program.

7. A PREWORKOUT SUPPLEMENT. What you want from a good pre-workout product is a more intense and focused training session with increased blood flow for a better neuromuscular response. Right now I'm using Grenade .50 Calibre. The first time I took it, I was around 15 percent body fat, yet my vascularity and increased muscularity were very apparent! It honestly felt like someone had pumped me up with two extra pints of blood!

A pre-workout supplement should substantially increase your intensity level, but without the mad rush, anxiety, and distraction that sometimes accompany it. When taking .50 Calibre you may find that you actually have to force yourself to take longer rests between sets, which is exactly what you want during the latter stages of the 12-week plan, when you enter the DTP phase.

FOOD PREPARATION: THE TRANSFORMATION SECRET

When the focus is to feed your metabolism and your muscles so your body will look toned, healthy, and lean, you absolutely need to eat every two to three hours. When you're eating this often, it can start to seem very time-consuming—if you aren't eating food, you are thinking about food, and if you aren't thinking about food, you are preparing it. With smart preparation, though, you can set the stage for a seamless transformation with a nearly automated system for fulfilling your nutritional needs. First, you have to stock your cupboards with a hoard of refrigerator containers. You should have some large enough to fit a meal, some slightly larger, to hold a couple of days' worth of vegetables, and the biggest to contain cooked carbohydrates and protein (separate tubs for each).

Like most of you, I have a very busy lifestyle that doesn't allow me to spend as much time in the kitchen as Gordon Ramsay, so I cook most of my foods in bulk. By doing this, I find that I can cook my weekly quota of nu-

SMARTER SERVING AND STORAGE

When it comes to food, it seems we can now say, "You are what you eat—and you eat what's nearby." Food psychologist Brian Wansink, the director of the Cornell Food and Brand Lab and author of *Mindless Eating: Why We Eat More Than We Think,* has conducted a lot of research on people's eating habits—enough to discover some pretty basic strategies for cutting out bad ones. One important discovery arrived when he and his team studied where people serve foods: when serving dishes were kept away from the dining area, people consumed 20 percent fewer calories. "Quite simply, it is a case of 'out of sight, out of mind,'" says Wansink. Instead, keep your serving dishes in the kitchen or on the stove so everyone has to go back to serve themselves more.

Wansink also suggests applying this same strategy to how you store foods. (Though I recommend clearing your kitchen of all unhealthy foods before you begin your transformation, you might have kids, a significant other, or roommates who don't want to clear out their food choices.) Keep all the healthy items at the top of the refrigerator or pantry—at eye level—and you're more likely to reach for those first. Also, big-box packages from stores such as Costco and Sam's Club can increase consumption, so transfer some to smaller containers and store the rest in the garage or closet. You can read more about Wansink's research at http://foodpsychology .cornell.edu/.

trition in two sessions. On Sunday, I fill my barbecue with fish, chicken breast, and some steak. I cook some brown rice in a rice cooker, and I have some sweet potatoes in the oven. For vegetables, I'll steam or sauté some frozen or fresh vegetables and make a big salad that I can portion out for a few days. Once everything is cooked, I separate the foods into large containers and refrigerate. I repeat this process once again on Thursday, which keeps my cooking time to a minimum. The only meals I like to cook fresh on a daily basis are my last meal at night and my breakfast, which I prepare the evening before I'm going to eat it. I find these freshly prepared meals at the end of the day rewarding; eating previously prepared meals throughout the day is satisfying and practical,

but you can't beat eating food right off the grill or out of the pan.

By preparing in advance like this, each day, I am able to portion the next day's meals from the larger containers into smaller containers so they're ready to go. That way, all I have to do when I wake up is warm my breakfast, eat, fill my cooler bag, and head to the gym for cardio and then immediately to the office. It's quick and convenient, and it leaves room for no excuses for me to go out to lunch or head to the vending machine. Success doesn't just happen; you must prepare for it.

You might find it a little difficult to adjust in the beginning, but as with most things, it will quickly become habit. The majority of people don't have a problem getting to the gym a few times per week; what really separates the good bodies from the great ones is attention to detail when it comes to food planning and preparation. I always say that you will find your dream physique in the kitchen, so I want to make a special note to guys here: don't think you're too manly to put on an apron and figure out how that stove timer works—it's time to get cooking. Not only is proper nutrition essential to creating your transformation, it's one of the most important parts of our lives, yet it's an area where so many people lack control. Use the strategies I've outlined for you to help create control and fuel your body with the vital nutrients it wants and needs the most.

KITCHEN RENOVATION

I want you to take a look at what's in your cupboards and refrigerator and start to weed these things out of your house before Day 1. I don't want to encourage you to waste food, so if you've recently stocked up with non-transformation-friendly foods, donate them to a local food bank or someone you know who's struggling. I want you to concentrate on creating a "transformation-friendly zone," which is especially important in the kitchen, where temptations can lurk in every drawer or cupboard. Remember to reposition any unhealthful foods or drinks below eye level to help prevent impulsive eating.

Once you've removed all the necessary foods, drinks, and condiments, it's time to stock up with new foods. When you hit the grocery store, stick to the perimeter, where you will find all the fresh produce and meats—stay out of the junk-food jaws at the center of the grocery store; lined with cookies, crackers, and ice cream, they'll snap you up, and you won't escape without some debris in your cart. Another tip: don't shop when you're hungry; hunger will drive you to make some bad decisions.

As you start to eat to advance your transformation, I want you to focus on your food as fuel and eat with intention. Eating with intention means having a new connection to your food and seeing it as something that has a specific purpose—you are eating to feed your cells and tissues, to boost your energy, to reward your muscles and joints for their hard work, and to transform your body from the inside out. By staying connected to the food you're eating and its purpose, you will make the transition to transformational eating much simpler and more enjoyable—and before you know it, you will have established a new eating lifestyle.

Cheers to your transformation!

A New Mom Discovers a NEW LIFE

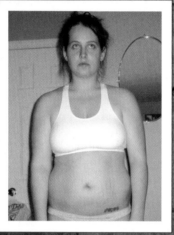

BEFORE

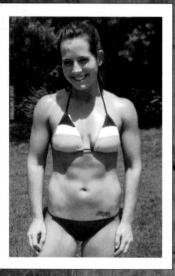

AFTER

After having her daughter, Charlotte Quillen discovered she loved life as a mom—what she didn't love was the weight she had gained during pregnancy and the way her body looked and felt postbaby. "I was in the worst shape of my life," she recalls. "And as a mother and a full-time student who also worked part-time, I knew I had to deal with the challenge of finding the time to get in enough training and eating."

She started off slowly, working in strength-training sessions when she could, but finally decided to become dedicated to her transformation. "Once I really committed to changing, I created a BodySpace profile and put myself out there so I would have a community of people to help hold me accountable," she says. "Having positive, like-minded people for support helped me stick to my goals and continue to push forward."

Charlotte discovered that one of the most important steps in her transformation was reevaluating her relationship with food. "I think this is the hardest part for most people," she says. "Food is fuel. You don't have to have junk food, even if you feel like you do—that is the food controlling you; I finally refused to be controlled by food."

Breaking bad habits wasn't easy, but she finally believed in her strength and ability to resist temptation—knocking down her doubts helped her make room for solid, positive new habits. "This is what my life used to look like: wake up late, eat a fast-food breakfast, smoke, drink Coke, play video games, eat fast food again (or junk food at home), smoke more, drink beer, waste money at bars, eat more fast food, and stay up too late—then repeat," notes Charlotte. "Now it looks like this: wake up happy, spend time eating healthy foods that fuel my body, play with my daughter, do some work, work out, spend time with my boyfriend—and go to sleep happy. That's a day I am glad to keep repeating."

She's actively tracked her progress with photos (posted on her BodySpace under the name beautifulgrace) and found motivation in seeing the changes and results show up in the images. "It's definitely a motivator for me," she says. She also discovered that it's not always enough. "Sometimes you need something outside of your own motivation to keep you going, and that's why having my BodySpace profile has been so critical in my transformation. There are members there who have added me to their list of people who inspire them—this really is amazing to me. I get messages daily from people thanking me for posting my before/after pictures, telling me I've motivated them to get back in the gym; this makes my day and makes me push even harder."

Charlotte has found a way to make sure she never misses workouts and suggests that others use the same strategy: "Plan them like you plan an important business meeting—it's not optional!" she says, offering a few other tips. "Keep your iPod handy, and if you don't feel the burn, add more weight. Ladies, you are not going to get bulky by lifting heavy weights—you are going to get toned and tight."

She maintains that a similar strategy has helped her stick with eating five to six small meals a day. "It's all about planning your meals like you plan anything else in your life," Charlotte notes. "The key is not to give up, because eating properly is an essential part of your transformation."

Now 60 pounds lighter and in a frame lined with toned muscle, she feels that her transformation has done more than just change her body—it's changed her life. "Everything has completely changed. I used to just coast through life, not take anything seriously, and definitely not take care of my body," she says. "Now I value my life more, take advantage of every opportunity, and strive to be a better person every single day. My commitment to a healthy lifestyle has also brought me and my boyfriend, Steve (read Steve's story next), closer together—he's been living this lifestyle for much longer than I have, and while he was patient with me, the way I was living before put a major stress on our relationship."

"The key is not to give up, because eating properly is an essential part of your transformation."

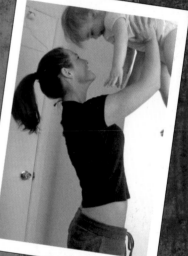

He Used to Wear Clothing
TRIPLE HIS SIZE TO HIDE

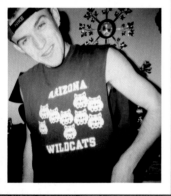

BEFORE

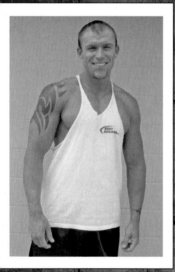

AFTER

With only 130 pounds on his five-foot, nine-inch frame, Steve Poynter felt he looked like skin and bones. Even though he had always been active, playing basketball, baseball, and football recreationally, his fast metabolism and naturally thin build kept him from ever really looking fit and left him feeling insecure about his size. "I used to walk around in clothing that was triple my size to help hide how small I was," he says. Then one day he walked into a gym and knew that from that moment on, things were going to change. "I knew that I would never stop going."

At first he worked out with no real structure, often overtraining and compromising his results. "I had no clue what I was doing," he recalls. He turned to fitness magazines first and pored over training articles to help expand his knowledge. "Then I discovered BodySpace and found this to be a great motivator in what I was hoping to accomplish," he says, acknowledging that with the motivation came an enhanced level of commitment. "There is no better way to stay focused than by logging into the site on a daily basis and looking at progress pictures, lifting stats, and training videos."

Steve, who is known as stevep78 on his profile, found that there were some obstacles to overcome during his transformation. "There was always something that made me think I could not achieve the look I was after," he says. "The biggest thing was to continue going to the gym—as the skinniest guy in there, I found it difficult to walk around what appeared to me as giants; it was very intimidating, to say the least."

He also found some resistance or lack of true support from those around him. "There are people who always want to keep you down and never see you succeed in anything, especially when it comes to body change," he notes. "There were always the constant comments like 'What are you doing? You're wasting your time.' Those are things you will always hear, but you are the one who has to keep the focus, drive, and determination. It's your body—make the change happen."

As he stayed the course and stuck to his commitments, an interesting thing happened: "All the negative talk went away and those same people became motivated to make a change as well." Steve was more than willing to help them begin their own transformation. "I started helping a couple of overweight friends lose some weight," he says. "I made up workouts for them, and through trial and error helped them get a healthy meal plan in order." A love for this process grew and eventually developed into a career: he now runs a business that provides other people with online personal training. "I couldn't be any happier than I am with how I look, and now I can help other individuals change their life through fitness and healthy eating." One of those people is his girlfriend, Charlotte Quillen (read her story on page 128).

His tips for a successful personal transformation include setting short-term, attainable goals first, then pushing yourself a little further each time you revisit your goals. Another key to sticking to goals: find a solid system of accountability. "A good tip for staying motivated and on track is to find an online source like BodySpace," he says. "You can always make friends on there and stay in touch with those with similar goals—you can push each other to do better.

"I also stress the point that everyone should feel in control of his or her own body. You control everything that goes into your body; you are the only one who can truly make change happen."

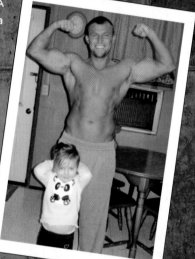

"You are the one who has to keep the focus, drive, and determination. It's your body—make the change happen."

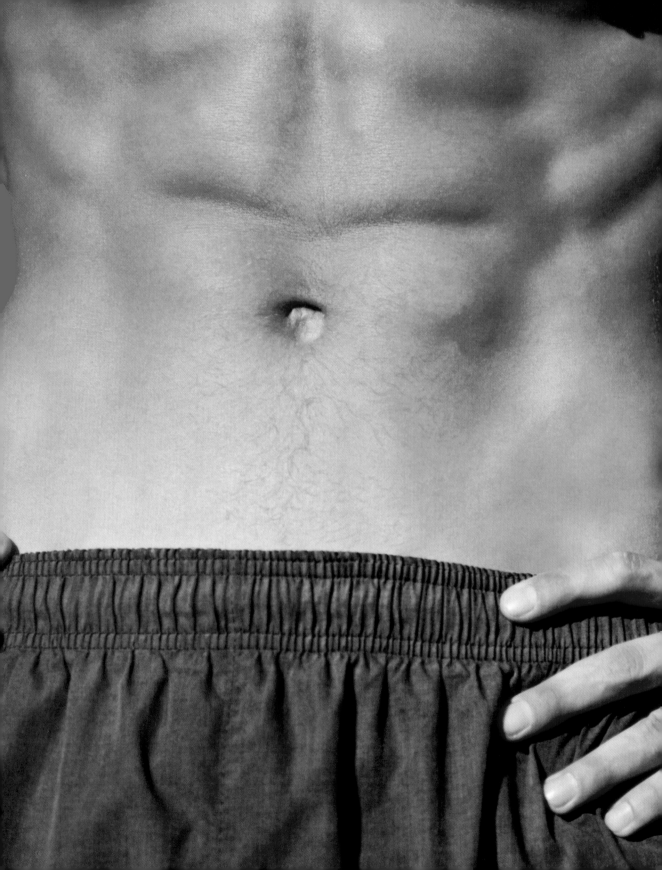

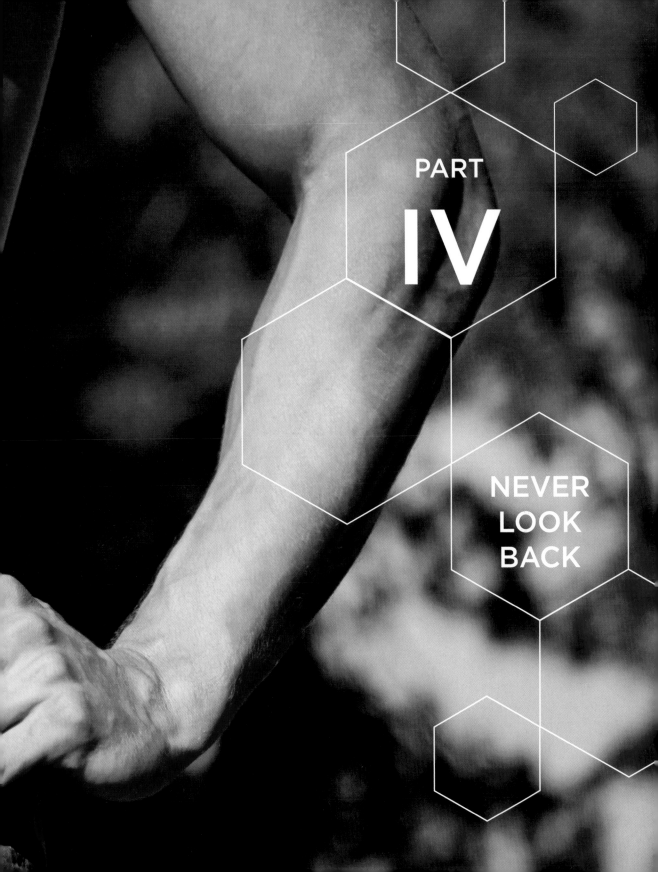

PART

IV

NEVER
LOOK
BACK

CHAPTER 9

Living with SUCCESS

I want you to do a quick exercise in time travel with me—a visualization that involves peering into the life of your future self. I want you to imagine seeing yourself as the person you've always wanted to be—the person who has finally erased the gap that existed between you and your ideal self. You have become the person you envied: the one who had more discipline or willpower than you, the one who created a profound change in his or her life—the change you thought you would never achieve. Those doubts are gone. You are living in your dream—and it's so much better than you could ever have imagined. Twelve weeks from now, this vision will be your reality; *you will have transformed your life.*

So now that you're there, is it time to drop the ball and return to your former life—the one filled with bad habits and low energy, a life in which you were nothing more than a passive participant just letting the days pass you by? I'm going to assume you're shaking your head no, which means you have answered correctly. You are absolutely not to let go of the progress you've worked so hard to create, but you are going to make some changes.

TURNING YOUR TRANSFORMATION INTO AN ENDURING LIFESTYLE

The reason some people "fall off the wagon" after they've completed a transformation is that they don't focus on creating new challenges. Remember how we created progress by strategically mixing things up in the phases of the Body by Design workout program? That was because your body adapts to workouts, and if you want to continue to create results, you have to modify the challenges to prevent plateaus. A similar thing happens to our brains and our motivation. By Week 13 will you have established new habits and connected to a robust and thriving motivation? Certainly, but

even the greatest athletes, the sharpest businesspeople, those who are perpetually at the top of their game have to rejuvenate their drive—in fact, they stay at the top because they are continually evolving and pushing themselves to new limits.

My first step for you, then, is to revisit your FLOW Chart. Hopefully you've kept your FLOW Chart nearby to help keep you on track and can easily return to it for review. Take a look at the goals you identified then and consider how true they are to the new you. Just to give you a little refresher: FLOW stands for Fixed, Limitless, Opportunities, and Weaknesses. Your fixed goal was about an outcome you wished to see in your appearance, and the limitless one was a long-term, intrinsic type of motivator (the other two, I think, are self-explanatory, but you can turn back to page 53 to review the FLOW system if needed).

When you've completed your transformation, I encourage you to make another copy of the FLOW Chart from the Resources section and identify your goals and weaknesses as you see them now. I myself am constantly redefining my own goals and personal challenges, and I find it essential to keeping me committed to my healthful lifestyle.

In the thousands of transformations I've witnessed and in those I've helped create, I've seen lasting success happen for those who've continued to stimulate their newfound active lifestyle and taste buds. This can come in the form of trying new things, such as training to run a 10K or giving a different type of diet (still with a clean eating foundation) a try. Upon finishing my most recent transformation, I decided to eat vegetarian for a month. I knew I needed to create another, smaller goal to keep my brain stimulated and away from thoughts of fattening foods and inactivity.

When you have worked so hard to schedule mealtimes and cardio and training sessions, to stay motivated and focused, it is easy to become depressed or lose momentum when you no longer have a specific goal, a daily structure, and a routine that releases endorphins (the feel-good substances that are released while you exercise). I call this the "posttransformation blues." The danger here is the lurking temptation of quick-fix foods that so many people turn to for comfort—you know them as comfort foods, and they're called that for a reason.

If you fall away from the structure of your commitments to good health and fitness for too long, it's easy to seek endorphins from other sources, and all too often they're in the form of unhealthy foods. The reason for this is that junk food, similar to a drug, can create a physical reaction in your body. Studies have shown that when we eat sugary foods, such as cake, chocolate, candy, and so on, our bodies can actually release endorphins, creating a temporary "high." Usually, while eating these foods we feel temporarily good, but then we sink into feelings of guilt and remorse and experience an actual physical depression. What's the first thing we reach for to make us feel better? More junk food. I'm sure you can see where this is leading—right back to the vicious cycle of dissatisfaction and disappointment and eventually back to the pretransformation doldrums. This is why it is important, now more than ever, to create another goal and become transparent with it to your friends on BodySpace and in your social circle at home.

EATING AND TRAINING RIGHT FOR LIFE

All too often, I've heard people say they were going to "eat this," "taste that," and then "eat some more" when their transformation had finished, and all too often their food choices have led them to consuming more than enough calories for a day in one meal. That's not how you ensure a long-term commitment to a healthy lifestyle, although you can make choices to include earned indulgences. Once you have completed your successful transformation, you can add in a cheat meal or day, but then you must continue to sup-

INSTANT INSPIRATION

"The difference between my life before and after my transformation is that now I am happy, motivated, and confident in everything I do."

—Peter*Dedicatedforlife

port those choices by eating well at all other times and training regularly. Once you have made a successful transformation, the last thing you want to do is unravel the sacrifices, the commitment, and the achievement you have worked so hard to accomplish.

Now is a good time to reintroduce some healthy fruits, grains, and fats, which will provide antioxidants and high-quality carbohydrates and aid in healthy hormone production. It's a good idea to introduce these into your weekly splurge meals slowly so that your body has time to rev up its metabolism and can adapt by burning off any excess calories it may be fed.

For the first week after your transformation, I recommend that you choose one meal that you have missed the most and have it for breakfast. Now, this shouldn't be waffles drowned in butter and syrup; aim to still make it a relatively healthy choice. Keep in mind that your body has adjusted to operating on food as fuel and feels best when nourished with high-quality foods, not empty calories. Trust me; if you go for that all-you-can-eat buffet or two-of-everything meal, you will not enjoy it or the food hangover it will leave in its wake. I love honey, Greek yogurt, almonds, blueberries, and pineapple, so I add these ingredients to my protein powder and oats in the morning. I like to have them at breakfast for two reasons. First, the antioxidants, dairy, and healthy fats make me feel so much better and alert during the day, and second, having them in the morning allows me to burn off the

calories throughout the day, which is especially important if I feel like eating a lot more than I should.

The second week is when I recommend you add in another healthful meal option. I enjoy a burrito with a scrambled egg, chopped tomato, and melted fat-free cheese topped with salsa. Again, this isn't something that is listed on the twelve-week eating program, but it is certainly healthful and will satisfy your taste buds without derailing your achievement.

The third week is when I like to add peanut butter and blueberries to my protein powder to make a delicious smoothie, but that is when I stop. For the first three meals (including a new meal every week), I have something that feeds my craving and tastes great, but it's still a healthful meal that doesn't provide too many calories. For the next three meals, I generally stick to the Body by Design eating plan. One of the meals on the weekend is when I splurge, but only if I feel like it. A homemade burger or spaghetti bolognese are my regular weekly vices when I'm not going through a transformation.

As far as training goes, that stays the same. If you want to maintain or improve your overall shape, keep your commitment to the gym at three times per week. You can begin the Body by Design workout program again, or you can find many other training programs on BodySpace. Starting with your first posttransformation week, you can slowly taper back on the number of cardio sessions you perform. Begin by removing two of your fourteen cardio sessions each week until you are performing around five sessions each week.

You certainly don't want to return to the way you were, so you need to make a commitment to a new lifestyle and a better you. On the other hand, you don't need to follow the Body by Design nutrition and cardio program as strictly as you did for the twelve weeks.

The same goes for cardio: don't immediately drop from fourteen sessions per week to five; this can cause an adaptation for the worse.

ALWAYS HERE FOR YOU

This book is your evergreen manual for transformational change. Return to it as often as needed to help you get back on track; follow the action steps I've outlined in the Four Pillars chapters to realign your commitments if ever you falter. The core concepts you've discovered in these pages will not go out of style; they're not based on a trend or passing fad but are rooted in proven science about human behavior and will guide you without fail.

"I NEVER WANT TO GO BACK
to the Sluggish Person I Used to Be."

Sarah Murdick decided she didn't want to be one of those people who just accepts changes to their bodies as part of aging. "Before I started working out, I would have achiness in my joints as I got out of bed in the mornings," she recalls. "I've heard people mention having the same problem, and they've resigned themselves to the fact that it's a part of growing older. When I tell them, 'No way!' they seem very surprised. My joint pain went right away as soon as I started exercising and watching my diet."

She began her transformation when her kids had grown up and moved out of the house. "I finally took stock of my life and decided that I didn't look and feel the way I wanted to," says Sarah, who describes life before her transformation this way: "At the end of an exhausting day at work, I would resort to eating 'comfort food' of cookies and other sweets. I was depressed and spent a lot of time just sitting in a chair in front of the TV. I wore loose-fitting, unflattering clothes, and I never found time to exercise." She knew life could be better.

Sarah, who goes by the name mermaid lady on BodySpace, took a gradual approach by first researching nutrition and exercise and talking to others about weight loss and training, then incorporating strategies for creating change. "I tried to remove as much of the unhealthy food from the cupboards as I could," she says.

Sarah's goal is to inspire and motivate others toward a healthier, better life. "I wanted other baby boomers, especially women, to believe that this was something that they too could accomplish," she says. "I wanted them to understand that our society has led us to believe that fitness is only for the young—and that this is simply not true."

One of the most important aspects of creating true change in her life was developing new habits, which she refers to as "the key to transforming your life through fitness." Here Sarah shares some of her top health habits:

► **Smart eating and supplements.** "I try to eat my fruit and starches like grains and potatoes during the early part of

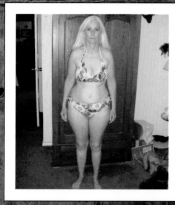

BEFORE

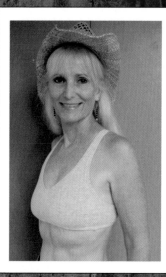

AFTER

the day. I use protein powder and supplements, which include glutamine, BCAAs, creatine, other amino acids, and vitamin supplements. And of course, I drink lots of water!"

➤ **Combating cravings.** "Chewing gum helps; and drinking a lot of water. There are some foods that I just can't have in the house, such as chocolate. If there is chocolate around, I will eat it all! You just have to know yourself and your limits. Keeping busy is the key to not obsessing about food—grab some herbal tea and a good book, and leave the kitchen!"

➤ **It all starts with you.** "Our actions have a domino effect with far-reaching consequences, for better or worse. My commitments to health have inspired my sister, who has been quite overweight most of her adult life, to lose over 30 pounds—and there's no stopping her now. She, in turn, is encouraging others to eat better and exercise."

Sarah's commitments to herself and her health have become a permanent lifestyle, one that has brought with it the unexpected gift of self-discovery. "Clean eating and exercising really helped to uncover the real me that was hiding for all those years," she says. "I never want to go back to the sluggish, dowdy-feeling person I used to be. I have plenty of energy to do my work as a massage therapist, to garden, and do other chores throughout the day. Plus, it's more fun to get dressed up and go out to social gatherings, and I feel a sense of increased confidence when meeting people for the first time. The biggest difference is that I am a happier person."

> "Clean eating and exercising really helped to uncover the real me that was hiding for all those years."

"I knew at That Very Moment MY LIFE WAS ABOUT TO CHANGE."

"My doctor said to change my lifestyle or die young," recalls Ed Cook of the moment that began his transformation. "I was told that my blood pressure, heart rate, sugar, and cholesterol were all borderline high, and that if I continued on the path I was on, I would end up with serious heath problems that would not only shorten my life, they would make my life miserable. I went to the gym that very day and joined."

Even though the first step toward changing his life was a physical one, Ed knew that if his commitment were going to be a lasting one, he would have to approach it from a more holistic perspective. "I discovered that all aspects of life need attention—spiritual, mental, emotional, physical—balance is key," he says. "Change isn't just about modifying your physical habits; you have to start with the foundation, not the roof."

Ed began shifting his thought patterns from ones that were self-defeating to ones with a more positive angle. "I believe that whatever you think becomes your reality," he says. "I really started to believe I could succeed, and I made the decision to choose a different path—I stopped feeling sorry for myself."

He also made an effort to surround himself with only positive people. One of the key steps in this effort was creating a BodySpace profile, which he did with the nickname oldsuperman. "Shortly after I had joined and filled out my profile, I was invited to join a forum for people over 35. Not only did I gain support and access to helpful information, most important, I have made lifelong friends."

A crucial part of his transformation was learning the importance of one vital strategy: planning. As a busy father of four and the owner of two businesses, both of which require travel, planning has proven essential to Ed's success. Here are some of his tips for making it all work.

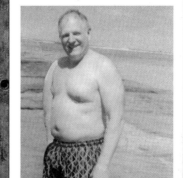

BEFORE

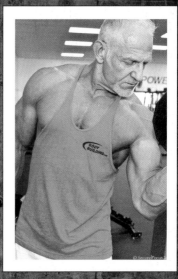

AFTER

➤ **Know your weaknesses.** "I love candy and sweets, and with four kids and lots of family activities, it was and still is unreasonable to think you can just remove bad foods from your life. There are birthday parties, weddings, family barbecues, Easter, Valentine's Day; I just had to plan properly. Fill your house with as many types of healthy treats as you can. I also bring my own food to parties a lot, things like low-fat and sugar-free desserts."

➤ **Be creative.** "I buy lots of variety when it comes to food. I prepare about three to six meals a day, depending on if I'm traveling. I buy meat in large portions, rarely frozen because I prefer fresh. I cook and prepare my food every two to three days and separate it into small microwaveable containers, which I'll put in my small cooler. I have also found that almost all restaurant chains will cook anything any way you like it."

➤ **Plan for detours.** "I always have a backup plan. Sometimes family or work will interfere with training or diet, so I always carry extra healthy food and snacks with me or double up training to make up for a missed session."

➤ **Don't be afraid to take control.** "You have to understand that this is your journey and be willing to accept accountability for your life. What helped was finding support from others who had my same goals and interests, which included getting a training partner."

At 56, and in the best shape of his life, Ed feels there's still room for improvement, and he works toward it with the help of a chain of inspiration he's tapped into on BodySpace. "I get a lot of messages from people asking questions and telling me I've inspired them, but I am the one who is inspired," he says. "I am grateful for the people there who have helped me see once again what's most important in life: giving, not getting."

"I really started to believe I could succeed, and I made the decision to choose a different path."

Conclusion: CONGRATULATIONS!

If you have completed your twelve-week transformation, keep reading; if you have not, return to page 86 and put your transformation into motion. I'd like you to think of this page as a gift you've saved for that special occasion—the reward or acknowledgment you receive after you've put in the hours of hard work, dedication, sweat, heart, and soul. I want you to have earned my congratulations because I don't issue the words carelessly. To those of you who have followed the Body by Design plan and accomplished a lifestyle overhaul, I say congratulations. You've stripped away layers of baggage, whether in the form of self-doubt, unwanted pounds, or negative social ties; you have achieved the extraordinary and reinvented yourself. Congratulations for choosing a different path—for choosing to truly live by treating your body as though it's the only one you've got. Be sure to thank yourself for that precious gift, because there are far too many people out there who overlook this simplest of truths.

And speaking of those people . . . your next step is to begin reaching out to them, because isn't the gift of a healthy life something you want to pass on? Start with the ones you love most and extend your reach as far as you can. Take the power and energy your transformation has bestowed on you and begin reaching out—even though you don't know it, chances are you've already begun to spread health around you, planting seeds of change with your enthusiasm and vitality (I'm sure it doesn't hurt either that you look amazing).

You may recall how I have talked about things spreading through people—from big, behavioral things such as obesity, to small things such as yawns and laughter. Your commitment to health and fitness does not stop with you—it *starts* with you and then it spreads, creating a chain of transformational change.

TOOLS FOR STAYING ON TRACK

If you haven't already created a BodySpace profile, I hope you at least check out the site, if only to drop by and let us know how you've done with the program. You can also join the Body by Design BodyGroup and connect with others who have followed or are following the plan. You'll gain access to member forums, connect with people with similar goals, and find plenty of peer support and feedback.

While there, I suggest you scan through some of our amazing tracking tools. As you stick with your commitments to work out and eat well, you can certainly continue to use the trackers provided in this book, but if you want to take things up a notch, you should see what we have to offer. You'll be able to download the customized Body by Design tracker that you can access by visiting www.body building.com/bodybydesign. Plus, you can upload dozens of progress pictures and check out other people's images and read their tips for success. Don't be afraid to send anyone a message asking how he or she did it—if you've learned anything from the success stories in this book, I hope it's that the people you'll meet on BodySpace are not only happy to help, they're waiting to hear from you because it fuels their own motivation.

Again, I want to congratulate you for your phenomenal transformation and thank you for letting me guide you through it. Remember: you are in control of your life, and you are now part of a movement—be proud of yourself and spread the word of fitness. Love life, don't just live it.

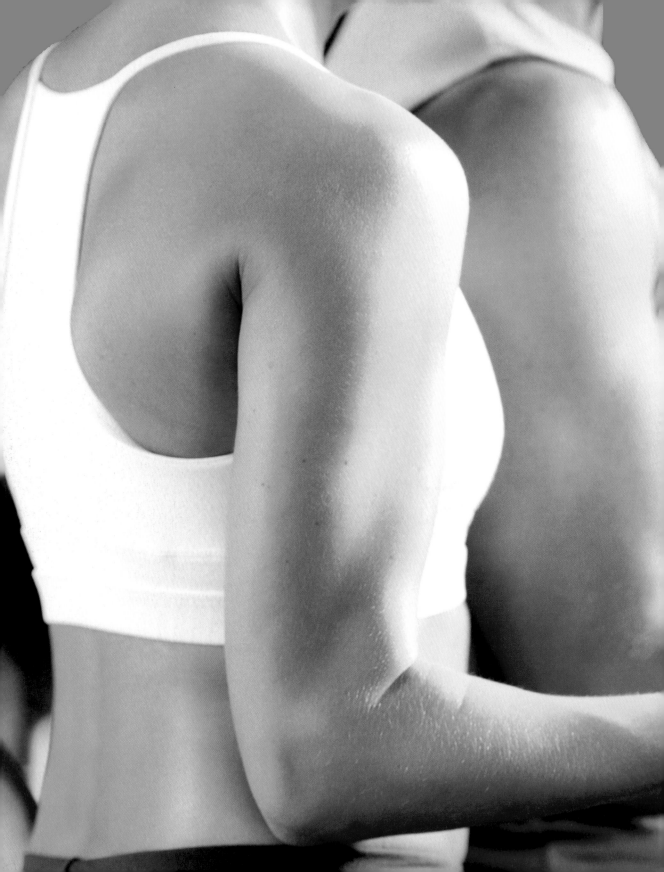

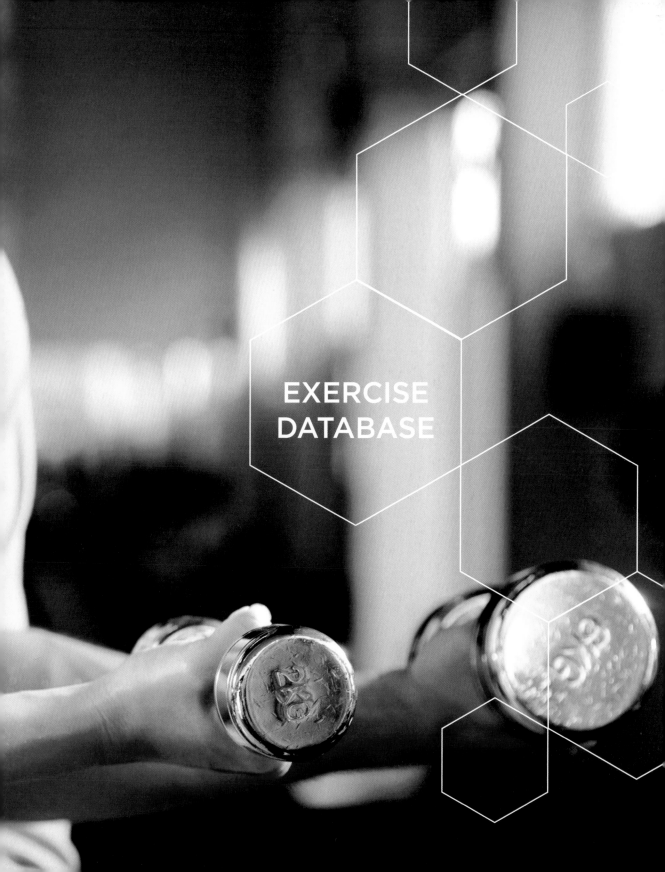

EXERCISE
DATABASE

BENT-OVER DUMBBELL ROWS

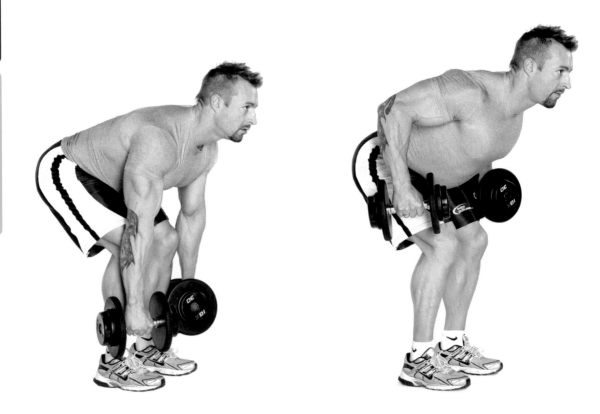

Start with a dumbbell in each hand. Bend your knees slightly and bring your torso forward. Keeping your back straight and head up, bend at the hips until you are nearly parallel to the floor. The weights should hang directly in front of you; your arms will be perpendicular to the floor. This is your starting position. Keeping your torso stationary, lift the dumbbells to your sides as you exhale, keeping your elbows close to your body. As you pull, squeeze your shoulders back and hold for a brief pause. Inhale as you slowly lower the weights back to the starting position.

DUMBBELL DEADLIFTS

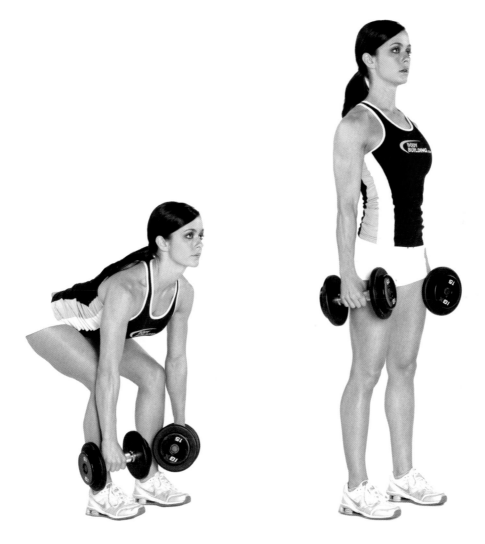

Place two dumbbells on the ground in front of you. Keeping your back as straight as possible, bend your knees, bend forward, and grasp the dumbbells, lifting them about six inches off the floor. This will be your starting position. Start the lift by pushing with your heels as you exhale and extend your hips and your knees. As you approach the standing position, pull your shoulder blades together and drive your hips forward. Inhale as you slowly return to the starting position by bending your knees and hips and leaning forward at the waist, keeping your back straight. When the dumbbells are lowered halfway down your shins, you are ready to perform another repetition.

DUMBBELL SHRUGS

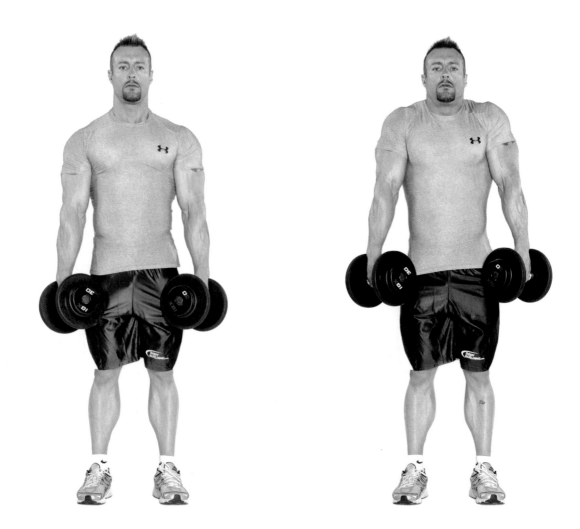

Stand erect with a dumbbell in each hand with your arms at your sides, your palms facing your torso. This will be your starting position. Exhale as you raise the dumbbells as high as possible by elevating your shoulders; keep your arms extended at all times and move only your shoulders up and down. Hold the contracted position for one second, then inhale as you slowly lower the dumbbells back to the starting position.

HYPEREXTENSIONS

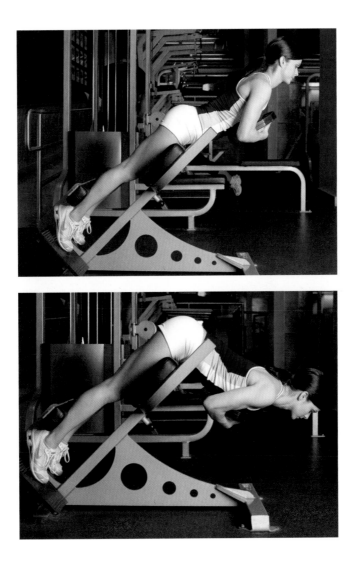

Lie facedown on a hyperextension bench, tucking your ankles securely under the footpads. Adjust the upper pad to allow you to bend at the waist without any restriction. With your body straight, cross your arms in front of you. You can hold a weight plate for extra resistance if needed. This will be your starting position. Bend forward slowly at the hips as far as you can while keeping your back flat. Keep bending until you feel a nice stretch on the hamstrings and you can no longer keep going without rounding your back. Slowly raise your torso to the starting position.

LATERAL PULLDOWNS

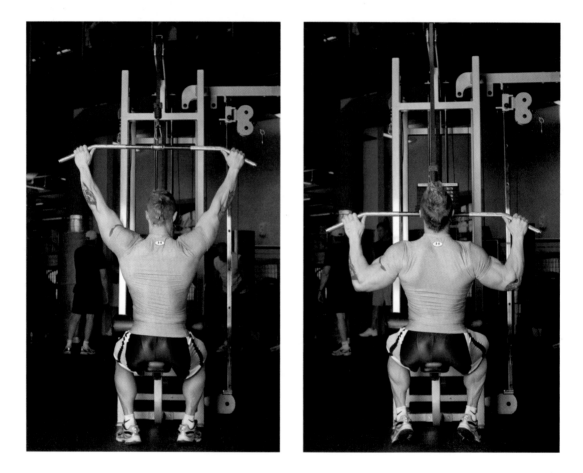

Attach a wide bar to the top pulley of a pulldown machine and sit down, adjusting the knee pad to fit snugly against your legs. Grip the bar wide with the palms of your hands facing away from your body. Lean your torso back slightly to create a small curvature in your back and stick your chest out. This will be your starting position. Exhale and bring the bar down until it touches your upper chest. As you pull the bar down, squeeze your shoulder blades back and down. Your upper torso should remain stationary during the movement, and only your arms should move. After a brief pause at the bottom, contracted position, inhale as you slowly raise the bar back to the starting position with your arms fully extended, feeling a slight stretch in your lats.

REVERSE-GRIP PULLDOWNS

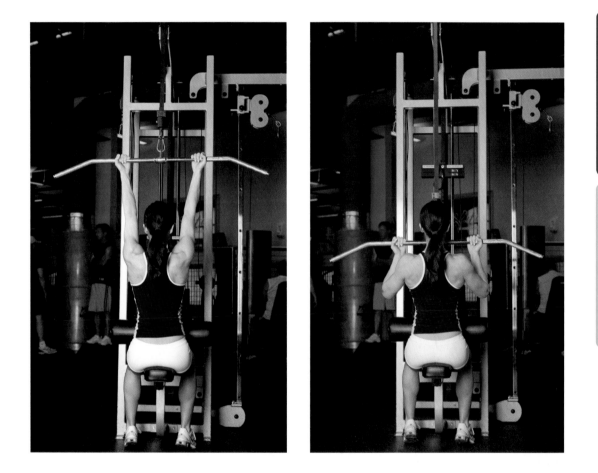

Attach a wide or cambered bar to the top pulley of a pulldown machine and sit down, adjusting the knee pad to fit snugly against your legs. Grab the pulldown bar with your palms facing your torso. Make sure that your hands are about shoulder width apart. Lean your torso back slightly to create a small curvature in your back and stick out your chest. This is your starting position. Now, as you exhale, pull the bar down until it touches your upper chest by drawing your shoulders and upper arms down and back. Focus on squeezing your back muscles once you reach the fully contracted position, keeping your elbows close to your body. Your upper torso should remain stationary during the movement, and only your arms should move. After a brief pause at the bottom, contracted position, inhale as you slowly raise the bar to the starting position with your arms fully extended, feeling a slight stretch in your lats.

SEATED CABLE ROWS

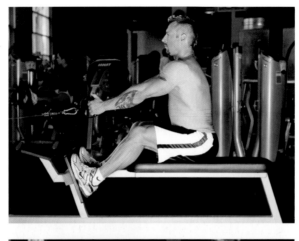

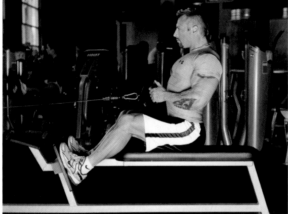

For this exercise you will need access to a low pulley row machine with a V-bar. (**Note:** The V-bar will enable you to have a neutral grip in which the palms of your hands face each other.) To get into the starting position, sit down on the machine and place your feet on the front platform or crossbar, making sure that your knees are slightly bent and not locked. Lean over as you keep the natural alignment of your back and grab the V-bar handles. With your arms extended, pull back until your torso is at a 90-degree angle from your legs; your back should be slightly arched and your chest should be sticking out. This is the starting position of the exercise. Keeping the torso stationary, exhale as you pull the handles back toward your body, keeping your elbows in, until you touch your abdominals; at this point you should be squeezing your back muscles hard. Hold the contraction for a second and inhale as you slowly return to the starting position. Repeat for the recommended number of repetitions.

BARBELL CURLS

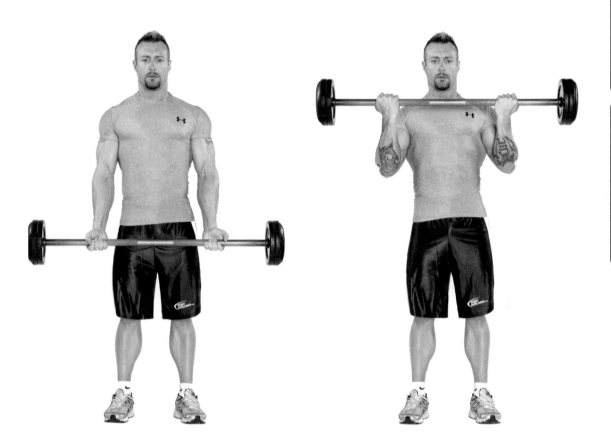

Stand up straight holding a barbell with a shoulder-width grip. The palms of your hands should be facing away from your body and your elbows should be close to your torso. This will be your starting position. Exhale and curl the barbell upward by contracting your biceps. Be sure to keep your upper arms stationary; continue raising the barbell until it reaches shoulder level. Hold the contracted position for a brief moment. Inhale as you slowly lower the bar to the starting position.

BICEPS CABLE CURLS

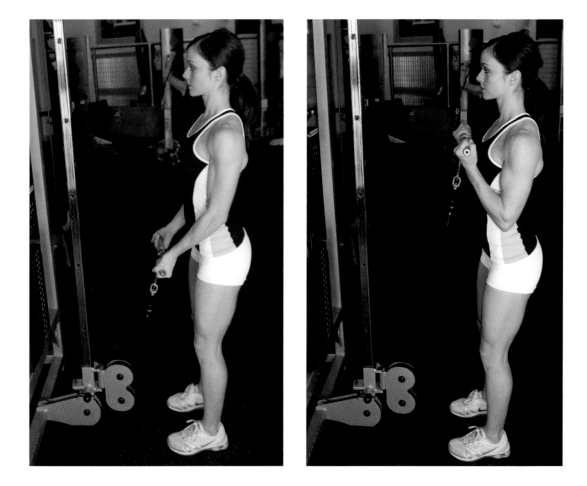

Attach a cable curl bar to a low pulley and stand facing the machine. Grab the cable bar with your palms facing up, keeping your hands shoulder width apart and your elbows close to your torso. This will be your starting position. Keeping your upper arms stationary, exhale as you curl the weights upward, contracting the biceps. Only your forearms should move. Continue to raise the weights until your biceps are fully contracted and the bar is at shoulder level. Hold the contracted position for a brief moment. Inhale as you slowly lower the bar to the starting position.

CONCENTRATION CURLS

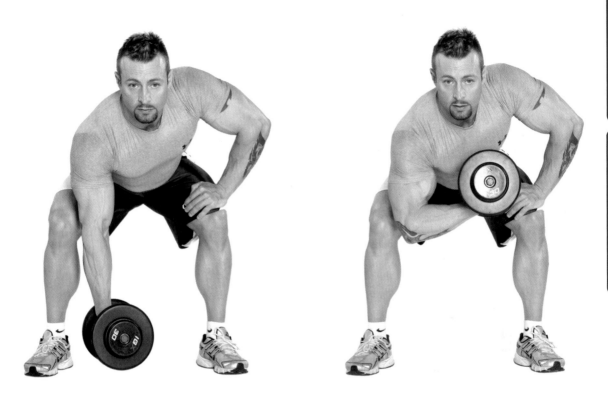

Bend over with your back straight and your legs slightly bent. With your right hand, grasp a dumbbell with an underhand grip. Place your left hand on your left thigh for stability and support. Now place the back of your right upper arm on the inside of your right knee. Your arm should be extended and the dumbbell should be lifted an inch or so above the floor. This will be your starting position. Holding your upper arm stationary, exhale as you curl the weight upward until it almost touches the left side of your chest, contracting your biceps. Hold the contracted position for a moment; inhale as you slowly lower the dumbbell to the starting position. Once you have completed the exercise with the right arm, do the same with the left.

PREACHER CURLS

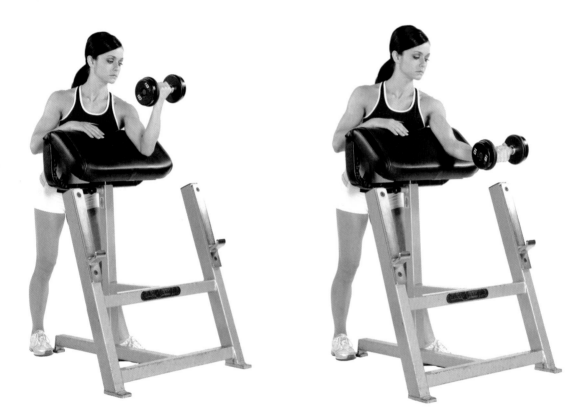

Position yourself on the preacher bench with a dumbbell in your left hand, your palm facing up. With your upper arms and chest positioned against the preacher bench pad, hold the dumbbell at shoulder level. This will be your starting position. Inhale as you slowly lower the weight until your arm is almost fully extended. Exhale, using your biceps muscle to curl the weight back up until your arm is fully contracted at the starting position. Squeeze the biceps and hold for a brief moment at the contracted position to get the maximum benefit. Once you have completed the exercise with the left arm, do the same with the right.

DUMBBELL FLYES

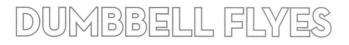

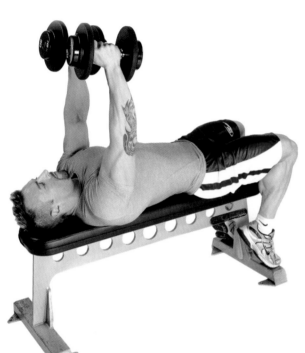

Lie on a flat bench with a dumbbell in each hand resting on top of your thighs, palms facing each other. Using your thighs to help raise the dumbbells, lift them one at a time until you are holding them in front of you, shoulder width apart. Raise the dumbbells up as if you're pressing them, but stop and hold just before you lock out. This will be your starting position. Keeping a slight bend in your elbows, inhale as you lower your arms in a wide arc, until you feel a stretch in your chest. Exhale as you return your arms to the starting position, squeezing your chest muscles. To perform this exercise correctly, imagine that you are hugging a large person, and focus on creating that same arc when lowering and raising the weights.

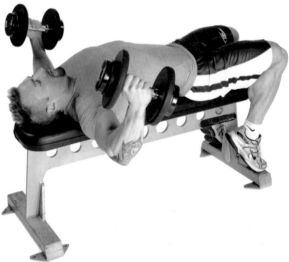

DUMBBELL BENCH PRESS

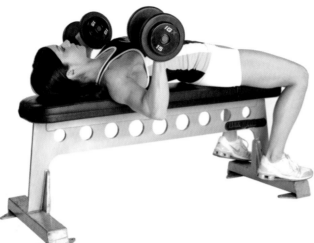

Lie on a flat bench with a dumbbell in each hand resting on top of your thighs, the palms of your hands facing each other. Using your thighs to help raise the dumbbells, lift them one at a time until you are holding them in front of you, shoulder width apart. Rotate your wrists forward so that the palms of your hands are facing your lower body. The dumbbells should be just to the sides of your chest, with your upper arms and forearms creating a 90-degree angle. This will be your starting position. Exhale as you use your chest to push the dumbbells up. Lock your arms at the top and squeeze your chest, then inhale as you return to the starting position.

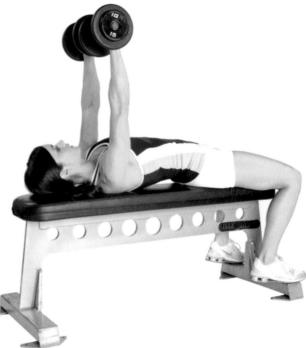

INCLINE DUMBBELL PRESS

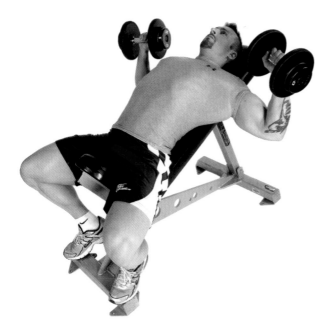

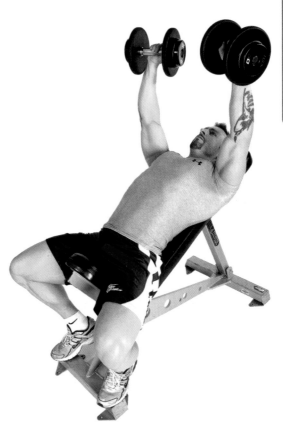

Lie on an incline bench with a dumbbell in each hand on top of your thighs, palms facing each other. Using your knees to help bring the dumbbells up, hold them out to the sides with your elbows bent at about 90 degrees, your palms facing toward your lower body. This will be your starting position. Exhale as you extend your arms and bring the dumbbells together above your head so that your arms are perpendicular to the floor. After a brief pause, inhale as you return the dumbbells to the starting position.

INCLINE DUMBBELL FLYES

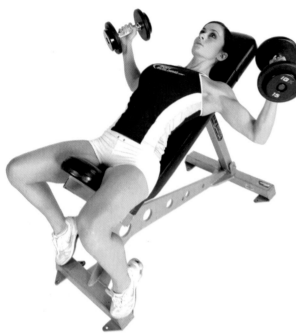

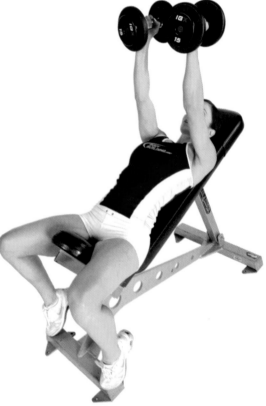

Lie on an incline bench with a dumbbell in each hand on top of your thighs, palms facing each other. Using your knees to help bring the dumbbells up, with a neutral grip hold them out to the sides with your elbows slightly bent. This will be your starting position. Maintaining the elbow position, exhale as you bring the dumbbells together above you so that your arms are perpendicular to the floor. After a brief pause, inhale as you return the dumbbells to the starting position.

STRAIGHT-ARM DUMBBELL PULLOVERS

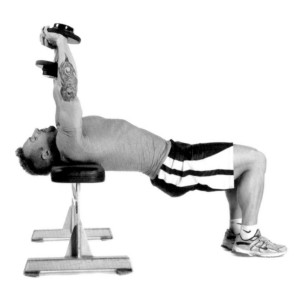

Place a dumbbell standing up on a flat bench. To ensure that the dumbbell stays securely placed at the top of the bench, lie perpendicular along the bench with only your shoulders on the surface. With your knees bent and your feet firmly on the floor, drop your hips just slightly below the level of the bench. Your head will be off the bench as well. Grasp the dumbbell with both hands and extend your arms up above your chest; your palms should be pressing against the underside of the dumbbell plate. This will be your starting position. Keeping your arms straight, inhale as you slowly lower the weight in an arc behind your head until you feel a stretch in your chest. Exhale as you return the dumbbell to the starting position following the same arc. Hold the weight at the top for a moment once you have returned it to the starting position.

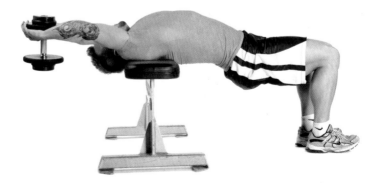

BENCH DIPS

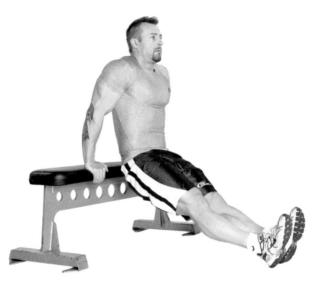

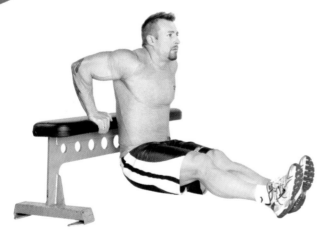

Hold on to the edge of a flat bench with your arms shoulder width apart and fully extended. Bend at the waist and extend your legs, your toes pointed toward the ceiling. This will be your starting position. Inhale as you slowly lower your body by bending at the elbows, forming a 90-degree angle between your upper arms and forearms. Exhale as you use your triceps to push your torso back up to the starting position.

TRAINER TIP: You'll want to keep your elbows as close as possible throughout the movement and your back close to the bench.

LYING TRICEPS EXTENSIONS

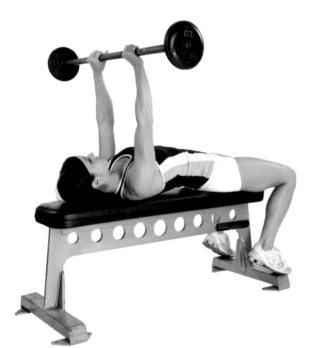

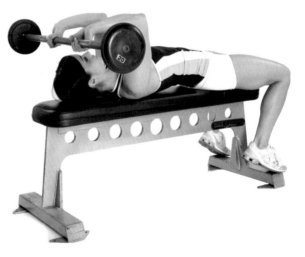

Lie on a flat bench holding a straight barbell with a medium overhand (pronated) grip. Raise the barbell in front of you and above the forehead at arm's length. This is your starting position. Inhale as you slowly lower the weight until the bar almost touches your forehead, keeping your upper arms and elbows stationary. Then exhale as you use your triceps to return the weight to the starting position.

ONE-ARM TRICEPS DUMBBELL EXTENSIONS

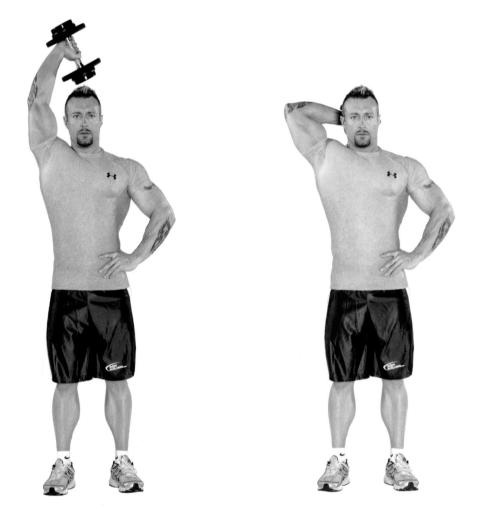

Pick up a dumbbell and stand up straight. Raise the dumbbell to shoulder height while with your other arm you hold on to a fixed surface, or place the other hand on your hip for balance. Extend your lifting arm over your head so that your whole arm is perpendicular to the floor and next to your head. Rotate the palm of your hand so that it's facing forward and your pinky is facing the ceiling. This will be your starting position. Inhale as you slowly lower the dumbbell behind your head while keeping your upper arm stationary. Using your triceps, exhale as you return the dumbbell to the starting position.

OVERHEAD TRICEPS CABLE EXTENSIONS

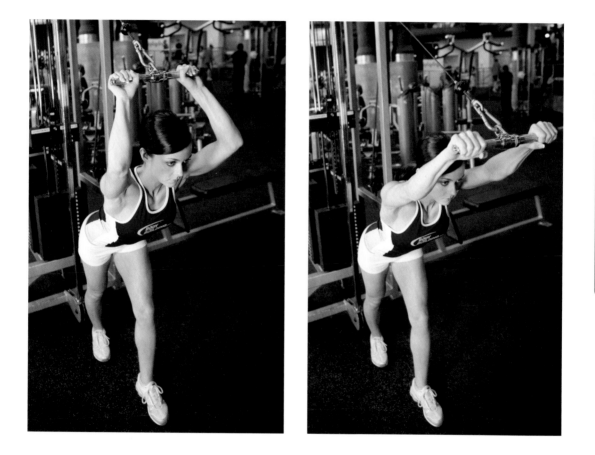

Attach a cable curl bar or a rope to the top pulley of a cable pulley machine. Facing away from the machine, grasp the attachment with both hands and lean forward, pulling your hands directly above your head. Your elbows should be close to your head while your upper arms are perpendicular to the floor with your knuckles aimed at the ceiling. This will be your starting position. Exhale as you slowly extend your arms until your hands are directly in front of your face while keeping your upper arms stationary. Once your arms are extended, inhale as you return to the starting position until your triceps are fully stretched.

TRAINER TIP: Your elbows should remain fixed throughout the movement.

TRICEPS CABLE EXTENSIONS

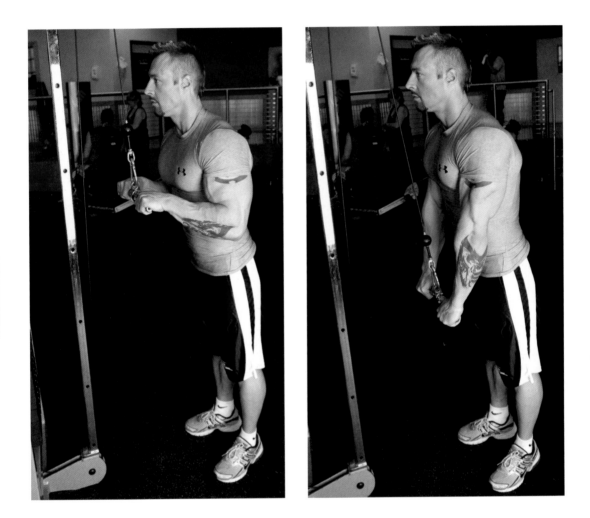

Attach a straight or angled bar to a high pulley and grab the bar with an overhand grip, your hands about shoulder width apart. Stand upright, leaning forward very slightly. Your upper arms should be close to your body and perpendicular to the floor. This is your starting position. Using your triceps, exhale as you push the bar down until your arms are fully extended. Your upper arms should always remain stationary while your forearms move. After holding for a brief pause in the contracted position, inhale and slowly bring the bar up to the starting position.

LEG EXTENSIONS

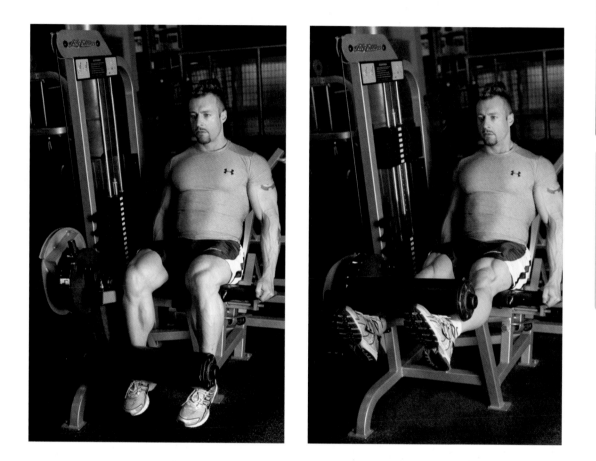

Choose your weight and sit on a leg extension machine with your legs under the pad, your hands holding the sidebars. This will be your starting position. Make sure your legs form a 90-degree angle between the lower and upper leg. Using your quadriceps, exhale and extend your legs while the rest of your body remains stationary on the seat. Pause a second in the contracted position, then inhale as you slowly lower the weight back to the original position, stopping right before the weight load touches the weight stack.

LYING LEG CURLS

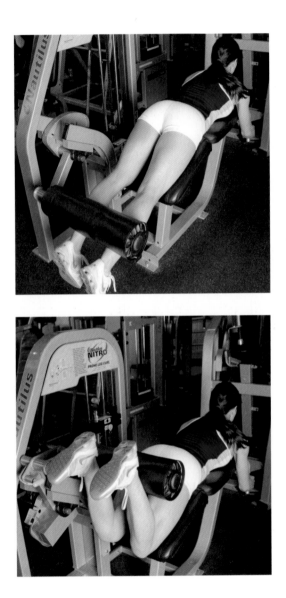

Adjust a leg curl machine to fit your height and lie facedown on it. The pad of the lever should be on the back of your legs, a couple inches below the fullest part of your calves. Keep your torso flat on the bench and ensure that your legs are fully stretched. This will be your starting position. Exhale as you curl your legs up as far as possible without lifting your upper legs from the pad. Once you reach the fully contracted position, hold for a brief moment, then inhale and bring the legs back to the starting position.

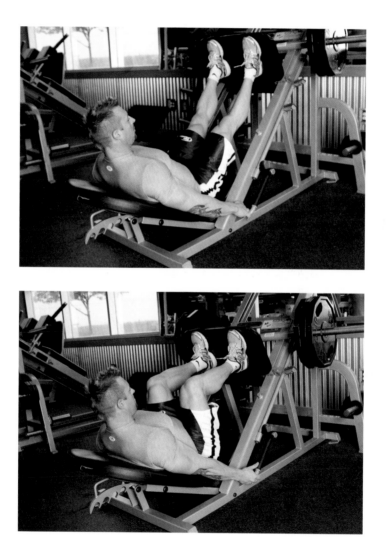

Sit down at a leg press machine and place your feet on the platform directly in front of you shoulder width apart. Lower the safety bar holding the weighted platform in place and press the platform up until your legs are almost fully extended in front of you; do not lock your knees. This will be your starting position. Inhale as you slowly lower the platform until your upper and lower legs form a 90-degree angle. Driving mainly though the heel of the foot, exhale as you push the platform back to the starting position.

SQUATS

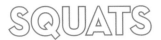

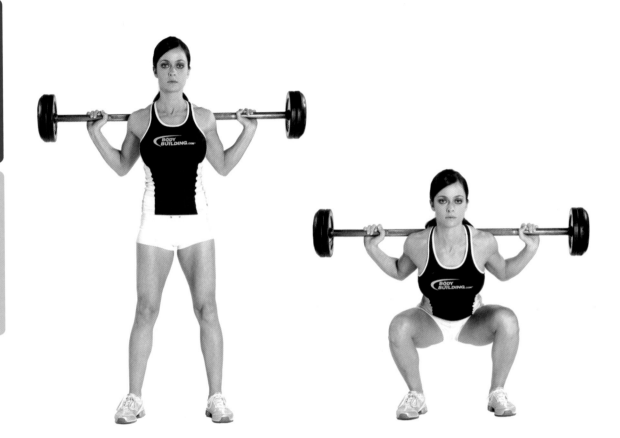

Set a barbell on a rack that best matches your height. Once it is loaded with your desired weight, step under the barbell and place the back of your shoulders under it. Lift the barbell from the rack by simultaneously pushing with your legs and straightening your torso. Step away from the rack and position your legs shoulder width apart with your toes slightly pointed out. This will be your starting position. Inhale as you slowly lower the bar, sitting back with your hips as though you were going to sit on a chair. Maintain the arch in your back. Continue lowering the weight until your hips and knees form a line parallel to the floor. Exhale as you lift the bar to the starting position, leading the movement with your head.

TRAINER TIP: As you squat, don't let your knees drift forward over your toes; keep them in line with your ankles throughout the movement.

SEATED CALF RAISES

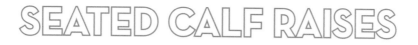

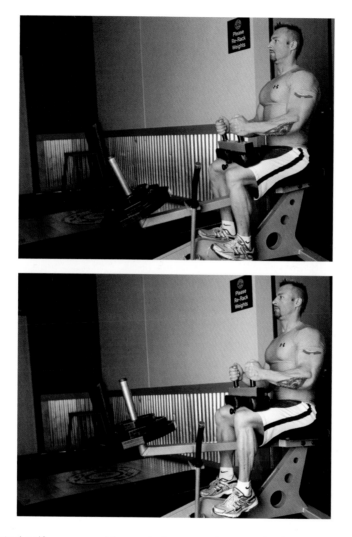

Sit down on a seated calf press machine and place your toes on the lower portion of the platform with your heels extending off it. Place your lower thighs under the lever pad, adjusting the pad to fit snugly against your thighs. Place your hands on top of the lever pad to prevent it from slipping forward. Lift the lever slightly by pushing your heels up and release the safety bar. Inhale as you slowly lower your heels by bending your ankles until your calves are fully stretched. This will be your starting position. Exhale as you raise your heels by extending your ankles as high as possible while contracting your calves. Hold the top contraction for a brief moment and then slowly return to the starting position.

STANDING CALF RAISES

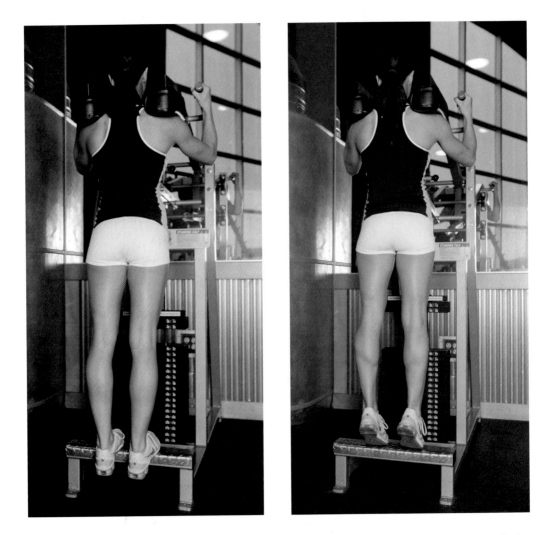

Place your shoulders under the pads of a standing calf press machine and position your toes facing forward. The balls of your feet should be secured on top of the block with your heels extending off of it. Push the lever up by extending your hips and knees until you can stand up straight. This will be your starting position. Now exhale as you raise your heels by extending your ankles as high as possible while flexing your calves. Hold the contracted position for a brief moment, then inhale and slowly lower yourself back to the starting position.

TRAINER TIP: Your knees should always keep a slight bend and should never be locked.

BENT-OVER REAR RAISES

Keeping your back straight, bend at the waist to pick up two dumbbells, your palms facing behind you. This will be your starting position. Keeping your torso stationary, exhale as you lift the dumbbells straight to your sides until your upper arms are parallel to the floor. Pause briefly at the contracted position, then inhale as you slowly lower the dumbbells to the starting position.

DUMBBELL SHOULDER PRESS

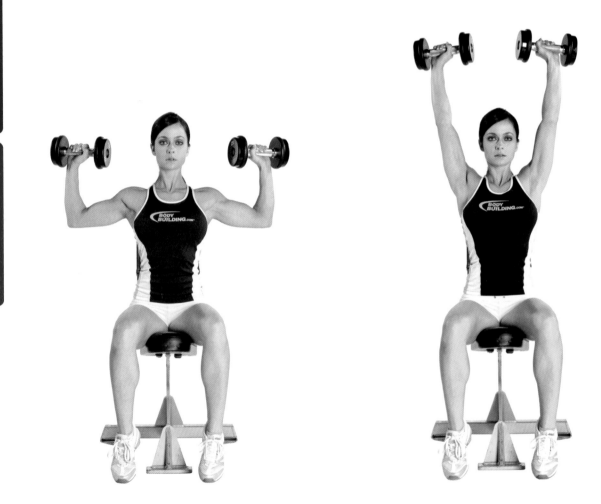

Holding a dumbbell in each hand, sit on a military press bench or utility bench with back support. Place the dumbbells upright on top of your thighs. Raise the dumbbells to shoulder height one at a time, using your thighs to help propel them into position. Be sure to rotate your wrists so that the palms of your hands are facing forward. This is your starting position. Exhale as you push the dumbbells upward until they almost touch at the top. After a brief pause at the top, inhale as you slowly lower the weights to the starting position.

FRONT DUMBBELL RAISES

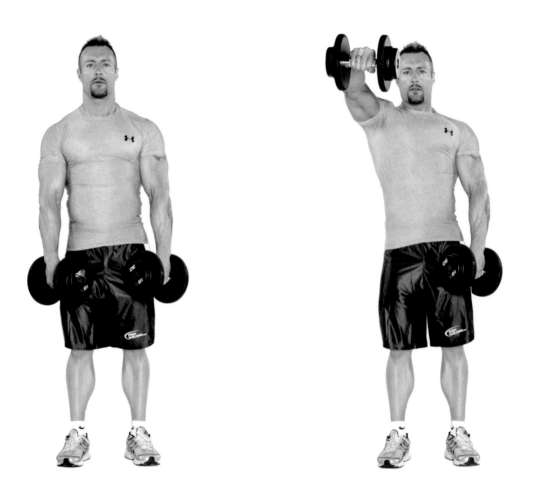

Stand up straight with a dumbbell in each hand in front of your thighs at arms' length, using an overhand grip. This will be your starting position. Without swinging, lift the right dumbbell to the front with a slight bend in your elbow with your palm facing down. Continue to lift it until your arm is slightly above your chest, and parallel to the floor. Lower the dumbbell slowly to the starting position, then repeat with the left dumbbell. Continue alternating in this fashion until the recommended number of reps has been performed with each arm.

SIDE DUMBBELL RAISES

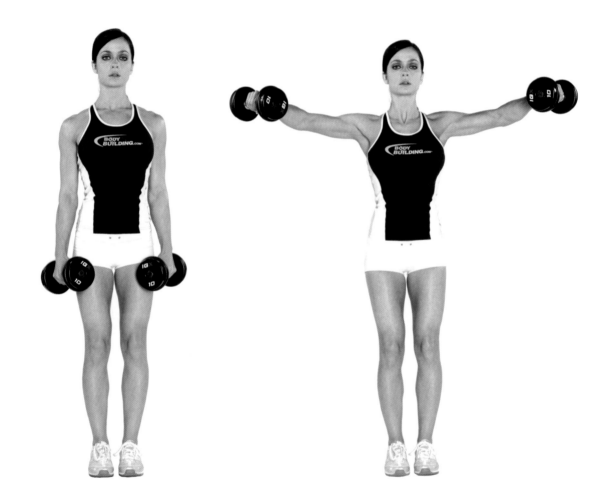

Stand up straight with a dumbbell in each hand at your sides, your palms facing you. This will be your starting position. With your torso stationary, exhale as you lift the dumbbells to your sides with a slight bend in your elbows, continuing to raise the weights until your arms are parallel to the floor. Your hands should be tilted slightly forward as if you are pouring a glass of water. Pause for a brief moment at the top, then inhale as you slowly lower the weights to the starting position.

ABDOMINAL CRUNCHES

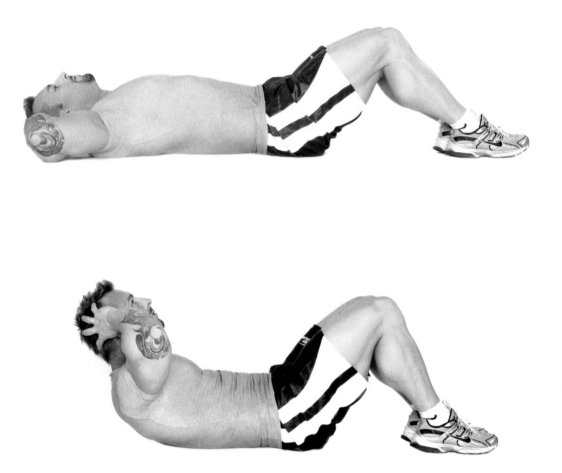

Lie on the floor. Place your hands on both sides of your head to support its weight and bend your knees with your feet on the floor. This is your starting position. Keeping your feet firmly planted on the floor at all times during the exercise, lift your shoulders and upper back up and away from the floor with your face pointing toward the ceiling. Although the range of motion is limited, exhale as you come up as far as you can, hold for a second, then inhale as you return to the starting position.

TRAINER TIP: You can increase the challenge of this exercise by adding a weight.

LYING LEG RAISES

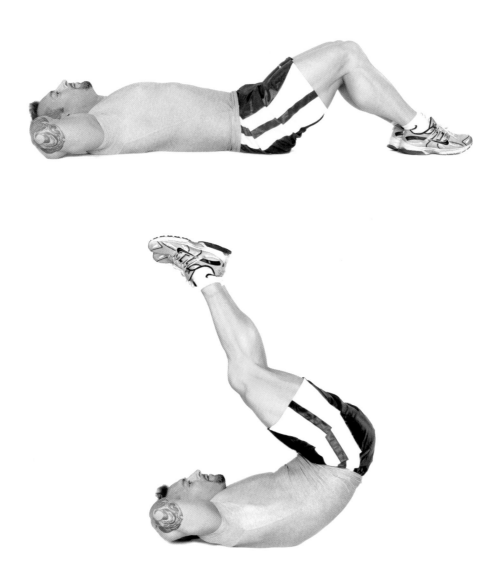

Lie on a floor, place your hands on both sides of your head, and bend your knees with your feet planted firmly on the floor. This is your starting position. Exhale as you lift your feet off the floor and tuck your knees toward your chest, extending the bottoms of your feet toward the ceiling while focusing on pulling your hips from the floor. Inhale as you return to the starting position without allowing your feet to touch the ground completely when they are lowered.

TWISTS

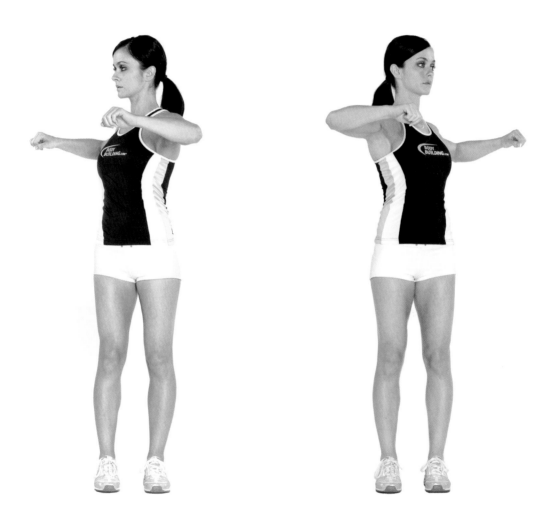

Standing with your feet shoulder width apart, your arms out to your sides and your elbows bent. Keeping your feet, head, and hips stationary, quickly twist your upper body from side to side so that your oblique muscles feel the contraction. Move from side to side only as far as your waist will allow you to go. Breathe continuously and contract your abdominal muscles throughout the exercise.

RESOURCES

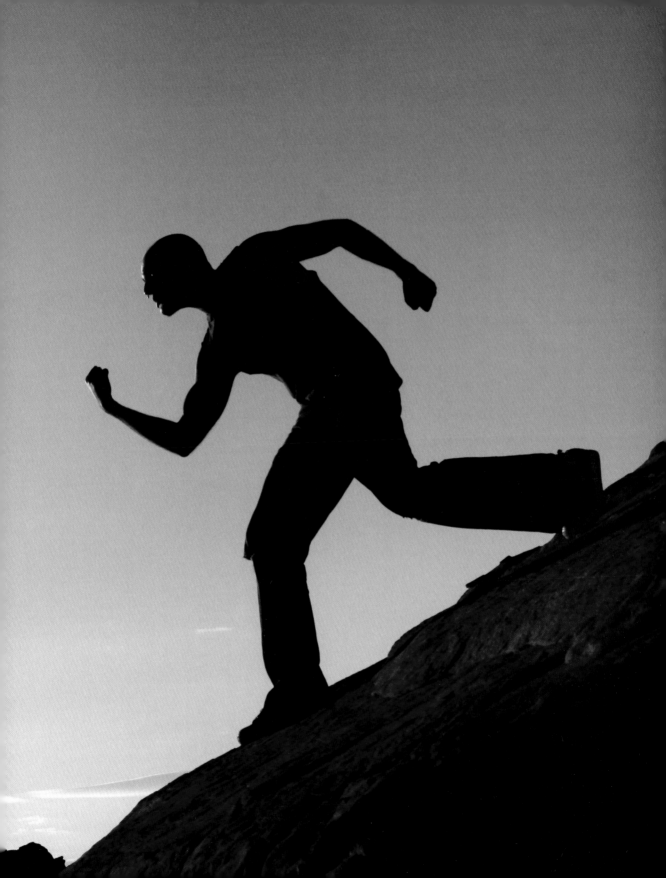

FREQUENTLY ASKED QUESTIONS

1. What if I miss a workout or a meal?

I know plenty of people will tell you to just let it go, "don't worry about it." Well, my advice is a little different. If you're don't worry about it, you set yourself up to accept excuses—and that's not a good habit to get into if you want to create solid new health habits. If you're careless about lapses, you risk falling back into your old habits. Now, this doesn't mean you need to literally punish yourself, but you should take inventory and see what factors are creating the holes in your commitment and make sure to patch them up.

Remember that awareness, motivation, and preparation are the keys to sticking to your goals. Revisit your goals, both public and private, to freshen up your awareness—you can't get to where you want to go if you don't know where it is. Give your motivation a boost by checking in with the people you've shared your

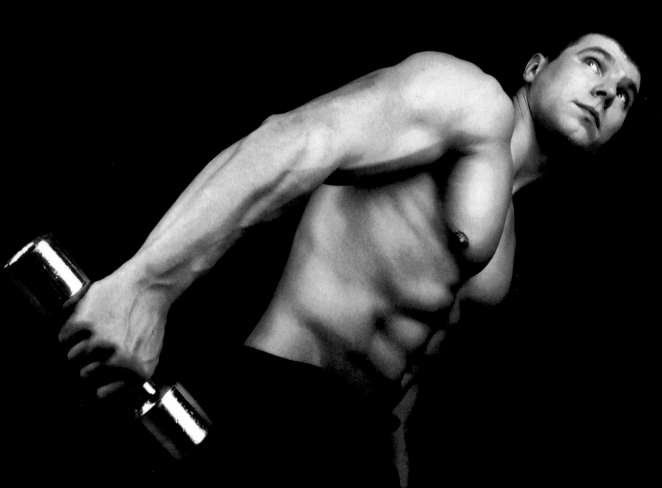

goals with; they'll be sure to offer words of encouragement to help get you back on track.

If you've missed a meal or workout and it's not due to illness or family emergency, chances are you weren't prepared. So ask yourself how you can be better prepared next time. Treat every workout as you would an appointment with an important doctor—write it in pen in your calendar (or add it to your phone or Internet calendar), and don't accept any excuses for missing it. When it comes to your eating, shop in advance for at least three to four days' worth of food and pack your meals into separate containers for the days you have to spend at work or school. Carry them with you in a cooler bag if you don't have access to a refrigerator during the day.

2. Can I drink coffee or tea during my transformation?

Yes. As I'm from Wales, drinking tea is as much a part of my heritage as being short and stocky and built for rugby. You can drink tea or coffee on this plan, even with a dash of milk, but that doesn't mean you can indulge in a caffe latte or cappuccino. If you prefer espresso, I recommend an Americano, which is espresso with a little water. Remember, the milk and sugar will add up, and caffeine acts as a diuretic, which can counteract your efforts to stay well hydrated—for these reasons, I suggest consuming caffeinated beverages in moderation. I normally have a weak coffee at breakfast and one before my workout, and I sometimes have a cup of tea during the day, usually if I feel hungry and

it isn't yet time for my next meal. I sweeten my coffee and tea with Stevia so I don't add calories, or I simply drink it without sweetener.

3. If I'm skinny and lean, can I add muscle and tone with this program?

Absolutely. Since you will consistently be fueling your body with muscle-building foods, you will begin to see muscle and tone develop. You will also begin to feel stronger after even one week on the plan.

4. I see you're telling lean people they can build muscle with this program; does that mean it won't help me lose weight?

This program will accomplish two things for you: it will help you build lean muscle *and* lose body fat. This means your percentage of body fat will drop and you will see your body develop a tight, lean look. Even if you don't see results on the scale quickly, you will see them in your measurements and in the way your clothes fit.

5. Can my teenage kids do this program with me?

Yes, with a few modifications. We've had several teenagers share their incredible success stories on BodySpace, and their transformations have been significant in shaping their lives.

Considering the soaring rates of childhood obesity, the sooner you can develop in them an interest in health and fitness, the better; this includes encouraging them to eat healthfully and properly fuel their growing bodies. Since they are still growing, I don't recommend focusing on cutting calories or eliminating certain foods such as fruits and dairy products, which contain valuable minerals and nutrients that growing bodies need. I also don't suggest taking the supplements I've included in this plan until the age of 18.

Check with your pediatrician just to be sure your child has the go-ahead based on his or her personal health history.

6. I don't have a gym membership—can I do this program at home?

Sure. Provided you aren't distracted by your home environment—kids, television, phone, couch, and so on—and you have a decent setup, you can do this program and get the same results as you would if you were visiting the gym. To follow the program exactly as it's laid out in this book, you will need to have a small cable setup at home; if you don't, you can visit www.bodybuilding.com/exercises to find alternative exercises that are performed entirely with free weights.

7. Do I have to take all the supplements you recommend to achieve results?

No. You don't have to take the supplements; in fact, you don't have to do anything I recommend—that is, if you don't want to get results as fast as others who follow the program to a T. Supplements don't replace a sound nutrition program, but they do add to it. What I am trying to say is that they will help you get results faster than you would without them.

8. I'm struggling to find people in my life who will support my commitment to a new lifestyle—what should I do?

Reach out and connect with those who have shared goals. Flip back to Chapter 3 for advice on how to break free from destructive influences and connect with new, positive ones. Looking for a place to start? Visit www .Bodyspace.com/bodybydesign; you will automatically gain a virtual connection to many of the top success stories in this book—including mine. Plus, you'll have instant access to hundreds of thousands of other people who were, or are, exactly where you are right now.

9. Can I drink alcohol during my transformation?

No. Alcohol, even antioxidant-rich red wine, has calories that do nothing to fuel your workouts and fuel only the fat deposits around your waist. Studies have shown that alcohol can increase cortisol levels, which promote fat gain, especially in the abdominal region—which should definitely be avoided when you are looking to trim down and show off a six-pack.

10. Do I have to do cardio?

Yes, cardio is a great way to spike the metabolism and provide energy for otherwise sluggish days (nonworkout days). Keeping your body fully revved throughout this program is essential to seeing optimum results. Not only is cardio great for heart health, it ensures that you get the most out of your strength-training workouts. You can't truly push yourself with weights unless you have the cardiovascular fitness to keep your body pumped with oxygen. And this goes for any guys out there who are thinking "Bigger is better." I know plenty of men believe that cardio will keep them from gaining muscle and keeping it on, but even if that's your goal, cardio is essential. If you fall short on cardio, I promise you, you will fall short on progress.

11. It's Day 1 for me, and I'm feeling really intimidated about stepping into the gym for the first time (or the first time in a while). How can I overcome those fears?

Honestly, most members of a gym are so focused on themselves and their own goals that they don't even notice that you are there. You'll see a lot of people working out with their headphones on, so they're truly in their own world. If it helps with your motivation and confidence, you can create a playlist of music that gets you pumped up—this can really help put you in the zone for your workouts. However, some people feel that music diminishes their focus, so try out both options and create the ideal environment for you. This is all about you and controlling your environment, so don't be afraid to customize it.

Consider this an opportunity for you to do what you fear and not fear what you do. As you begin to overcome your doubts about working out, you'll find increased courage and confidence in other areas of your life. For example, I hate public speaking, but I knew that when this

transformational book was published, I would have to hit the road and start talking to people just like you about it. I was excited because I'm passionate about it and I think it is truly going to change people's lives, but it also brought up an old fear of mine. So I volunteered to speak on stage at a big expo to help me get over my jitters—and I think having just gone through my own personal transformation helped me work up the courage to even get up there in the first place. I felt so much better at the end and relieved that I had achieved another goal—that first step broke down my fear and allowed my confidence to grow.

Following the Body by Design plan is going to change *your* life, so take the first step toward overcoming your fears by taking the plunge into your first workout; every one after that will be a little bit easier.

12. How should I keep track of my results? Should I use the scale or take measurements or pictures?

I find that pictures are one of the best ways to see how your body is changing. Many of our BodySpace success stories have taken weekly pictures and find that this is an exciting way to create a visual story of their transformation. Pictures also help you start to see where you may need to be working a little bit harder—photographs don't lie, so if you've been slacking during your leg workouts, for example, you'll see it right in front of your face. You can create your own BodySpace to upload up to twenty-five photos at a time or simply create a folder on your own computer where you can store images from each week.

13. I really want six-pack abs—can't I just do tons of crunches to get them?

You get your abs in the kitchen, not in the gym doing crunches. Without removing the layer of fat that is covering your abdominals through proper attention to nutrition, cardio, and weight training, you will never see your abs, which, even though you don't know it, are already there just waiting to be revealed. All you have to do is remove the cushion of fat and you'll make them visible!

14. Why can't I eat whatever I want since I'm working out and doing cardio?

Cardio is going to burn off only some of the calories you are eating before tapping into the ones you already have stored in your body. Fueling your body with unsuitable calorie sources will result in unsuitable results. Plus, you are eating very strategically to fuel your workouts; don't cut back on your potential by eating useless calories.

15. Am I going to be really sore? If so, what can I do to alleviate soreness or prevent it?

In the beginning, you will likely be quite sore. When you are training, you are tearing muscle fibers, but this is essential to creating progressive results. The more stress you increasingly place on your muscles, the more they tear down, being rebuilt as stronger and shapelier muscles. To help ease soreness, make sure you're taking the supplements glutamine, protein, and Vitargo after your workouts to assist with immediate recovery. Also, make sure you eat protein every two to three hours. If necessary, try a warm bath with Epsom salts to increase blood flow to your muscles and improve their elasticity.

16. I'm a woman, and I've always heard that lots of reps with light weights is the way to go. Is this true?

It's true if you don't want to change your body. When you lift light weights for a lot of reps, you may tire your muscles out, but you will not change them. Simply put, you have to challenge the muscle tissue on your body and add new lean muscle to create tone and give your body definition and shape. If you want to look great in a swimsuit or slip right into those favorite jeans, stop wasting your time with tiny little dumbbells—it's time for a true transformation.

17. I'm experienced with weight training and want to know if this program will still create results for me.

Yes, it will. I have been training for ten years now, and I am using this program as I write. I have gotten into the best shape of my life by using it and by staying consistent day in and day out.

18. If I have more questions as I go, where can I find answers?

Visit www.bodyspace.com, and you will be able to connect with other members following this very same plan by joining the Body by Design BodyGroup.

BREAKTHROUGH BUNDLE

Use the trackers and tools included in the following pages to define and document your goals and monitor your daily eating and workouts.

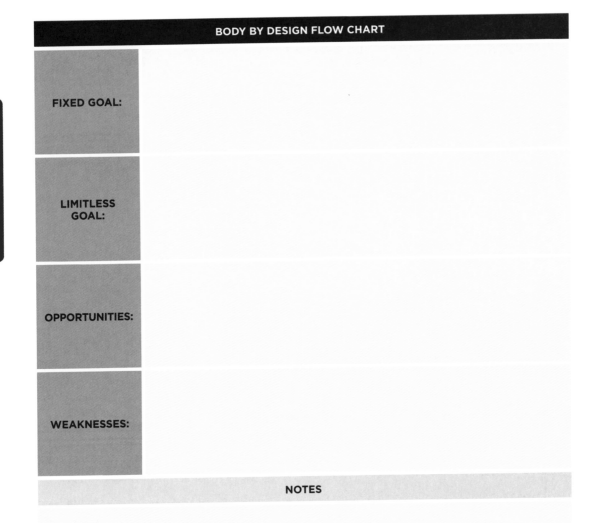

BODY BY DESIGN FLOW CHART

FIXED GOAL:	
LIMITLESS GOAL:	
OPPORTUNITIES:	
WEAKNESSES:	

NOTES

Phase 1, Day 1: Back, Upper Traps, and Biceps

DAY 1

Date:
Day _____ of 35

A.M. Cardio (20 minutes) ❑

EXERCISE	SET 1: TR	WEIGHT/ AR	SET 2: TR	WEIGHT/ AR	SET 3: TR	WEIGHT/ AR	SET 4: TR	WEIGHT/ AR
Lateral Pulldowns	15		15		15			
Seated Cable Rows	15		15		15			
Dumbbell Shrugs	15		15		15			
Hyperextensions	12		12		12			
Biceps Cable Curls	15		15		15		15	
Concentration Curls	15		15		15		15	

Phase 1, Day 2: Cardio and Upper Abdominals

DAY 2

Date:
Day _____ of 35

A.M. Cardio (20 minutes) ❑
P.M. Cardio (20 minutes) ❑

EXERCISE	SET 1: TR	AR	SET 2: TR	AR	SET 3: TR	AR	SET 4: TR	AR
Abdominal Crunches	20		20		20			

NOTES

_____

_____

_____

_____

_____

Phase 1, Day 3: Chest and Triceps

DAY 3

Date:
Day _____ of 35

A.M. Cardio (20 minutes) ❑

EXERCISE	SET 1: TR	WEIGHT/ AR	SET 2: TR	WEIGHT/ AR	SET 3: TR	WEIGHT/ AR	SET 4: TR	WEIGHT/ AR
Dumbbell Flyes	15		15		15			
Dumbbell Bench Press	15		15		15			
Incline Dumbbell Flyes	15		15		15			
Triceps Cable Extensions	15		15		15			
Bench Dips	15		15		15			
Overhead Triceps Cable Extensions	15		15		15			

Phase 1, Day 4: Cardio and Lower Abdominals

DAY 4

Date:
Day _____ of 28

A.M. Cardio (20 minutes) ❑
P.M. Cardio (20 minutes) ❑

EXERCISE	SET 1: TR	AR	SET 2: TR	AR	SET 3: TR	AR	SET 4: TR	AR
Lying Leg Raises	20		20		20			

NOTES

_____
_____
_____
_____
_____

DAY 5

Phase 1, Day 5: Shoulders and Legs

Date:
Day _____ of 35

A.M. Cardio (20 minutes) ❏

EXERCISE	SET 1: TR	WEIGHT/ AR	SET 2: TR	WEIGHT/ AR	SET 3: TR	WEIGHT/ AR	SET 4: TR	WEIGHT/ AR
Side Dumbbell Raises	15		15		15			
Front Dumbbell Raises	15		15		15			
Dumbbell Shoulder Press	15		15		15			
Leg Extensions	20		20		20			
Lying Leg Curls	15		15		15			
Leg Press	15		15		15			
Standing Calf Raises	15		15		15			

DAY 6

Phase 1, Day 6: Cardio

Date:
Day _____ of 35

A.M. Cardio (20 minutes) ❏
P.M. Cardio (20 minutes) ❏

DAY 7

Phase 1, Day 7: Cardio

Date:
Day _____ of 35

A.M. Cardio (20 minutes) ❏
P.M. Cardio (20 minutes) ❏

NOTES

_____
_____
_____
_____
_____

Key: TR=Target Reps; AR=Actual Reps

Phase 2, Day 1: Back and Biceps

DAY 1

Date:
Day _____ of 28

A.M. Cardio (25 minutes) ❑

EXERCISE	SET 1: TR	WEIGHT/ AR	SET 2: TR	WEIGHT/ AR	SET 3: TR	WEIGHT/ AR	SET 4: TR	WEIGHT/ AR	SET 5: TR	WEIGHT/ AR
Lateral Pulldowns	10		10		10		10			
Reverse-grip Pulldowns	10		10		10		10			
Bent-over Dumbbell Rows	10		10		10		10			
Dumbbell Deadlifts	10		10		10		10			
Dumbbell Shrugs	10		10		10					
Barbell Curls	10		10		10		10		10	
Preacher Curls	10		10		10		10		10	

Phase 2, Day 2: Cardio, Upper Abdominals, and Cardio Plus

DAY 2

Date:
Day _____ of 28

A.M. Cardio (25 minutes) ❑
P.M. Cardio (25 minutes) ❑

EXERCISE	SET 1: TR	AR	SET 2: TR	AR	SET 3: TR	AR	SET 4: TR	AR
A.M.: Abdominal Crunches	To failure		To failure		To failure			
P.M. PLUS: Twists	75/ side							

NOTES

_____
_____
_____
_____
_____

RESOURCES

Phase 2, Day 3: Chest and Triceps

Date:
Day _____ of 28

A.M. Cardio (25 minutes) ❑

EXERCISE	SET 1: TR	WEIGHT/ AR	SET 2: TR	WEIGHT/ AR	SET 3: TR	WEIGHT/ AR	SET 4: TR	WEIGHT/ AR	SET 5: TR	WEIGHT/ AR
Dumbbell Bench Press	10		10		10		10			
Straight-arm Dumbbell Pullovers	10		10		10		10			
Incline Dumbbell Press	10		10		10		10			
Incline Dumbbell Flyes	10		10		10		10			
Bench Dips	10		10		10		10			
Triceps Cable Extensions	10		10		10		10			
One-arm Triceps Dumbbell Extenions	10		10		10		10			

Phase 2, Day 4: Cardio, Upper Abdominals, and Cardio Plus

Date:
Day _____ of 28

A.M. Cardio (25 minutes) ❑
P.M. Cardio (25 minutes) ❑

EXERCISE	SET 1: TR	AR	SET 2: TR	AR	SET 3: TR	AR	SET 4: TR	AR
A.M.: Lying Leg Raises	20		20		20			
P.M. PLUS: Twists	75/ side							

_____
_____
_____
_____
_____

Phase 2, Day 5: Shoulder and Legs

Date:
Day _____ of 28

A.M. Cardio (25 minutes) ❑

EXERCISE	SET 1: TR	WEIGHT/ AR	SET 2: TR	WEIGHT/ AR	SET 3: TR	WEIGHT/ AR	SET 4: TR	WEIGHT/ AR	SET 5: TR	WEIGHT/ AR
Dumbbell Shoulder Press	10		10		10		10			
Bent-over Rear Raises	10		10		10		10			
Side Dumbbell Raises	10		10		10		10			
Front Dumbbell Raises	10		10		10		10			
Squats	20		20		20					
Leg Extensions	20		20		20					
Lying Leg Curls	15		15		15					
Leg Press	15		15		15					
Standing Calf Raises	10		10		10					
Seated Calf Raises	20		20		20					

Phase 2, Days 6: Cardio and Cardio Plus

Date:
Day _____ of 28

A.M. Cardio (25 minutes) ❑
P.M. Cardio (25 minutes) ❑

EXERCISE	SET 1: TR	AR	SET 2: TR	AR	SET 3: TR	AR	SET 4: TR	AR
P.M. PLUS: Twists	75/ side							

Phase 2, Days 7: Cardio and Cardio Plus

Date:
Day _____ of 28

A.M. Cardio (25 minutes) ❑
P.M. Cardio (25 minutes) ❑

EXERCISE	SET 1: TR	AR	SET 2: TR	AR	SET 3: TR	AR	SET 4: TR	AR
P.M. PLUS: Twists	75/ side							

_____
_____
_____
_____

Key: TR=Target Reps; AR=Actual Reps

BODY BY DESIGN DTP PHASE WORKOUT TRACKER

Phase 3, Day 1: Chest and Back

Date:
Day _____ of 21

A.M. Cardio (30 minutes) ❑

	EXERCISE 1	EXERCISE 2		EXERCISE 1	EXERCISE 2
	Dumbbell Bench Press	Bent-over Dumbbell Rows		Dumbbell Bench Press	Bent-over Dumbbell Rows
Set 1: TR	50	50	Set 7: TR	5	5
Weight/AR			Weight/AR		
Set 2: TR	40	40	Set 8: TR	10	10
Weight/AR			Weight/AR		
Set 3: TR	30	30	Set 9: TR	20	20
Weight/AR			Weight/AR		
Set 4: TR	20	20	Set 10: TR	30	30
Weight/AR			Weight/AR		
Set 5: TR	10	10	Set 11: TR	40	40
Weight/AR			Weight/AR		
Set 6: TR	5	5	Set 12: TR	50	50
Weight/AR			Weight/AR		

Phase 3, Day 2: Cardio, Upper and Lower Abdominals, and Cardio Plus

Date:
Day _____ of 21

A.M. Cardio (30 minutes) ❑
P.M. Cardio (30 minutes) ❑

EXERCISE	SET 1: TR	AR	SET 2: TR	AR	SET 3: TR	AR	SET 4: TR	AR
A.M.: Lying Leg Raises	25		25		25			
A.M.: Abdominal Crunches	25		25		25			
P.M. PLUS: Twists	75/side							

NOTES

_____

_____

_____

_____

_____

Phase 3, Day 3: Biceps and Triceps

Date:
Day _____ of 21

A.M. Cardio (30 minutes) ❑

	EXERCISE 1	EXERCISE 2		EXERCISE 1	EXERCISE 2
	Barbell Curls	Lying Triceps Extensions		Barbell Curls	Lying Triceps Extensions
Set 1: TR	50	50	Set 7: TR	5	5
Weight/AR			Weight/AR		
Set 2: TR	40	40	Set 8: TR	10	10
Weight/AR			Weight/AR		
Set 3: TR	30	30	Set 9: TR	20	20
Weight/AR			Weight/AR		
Set 4: TR	20	20	Set 10: TR	30	30
Weight/AR			Weight/AR		
Set 5: TR	10	10	Set 11: TR	40	40
Weight/AR			Weight/AR		
Set 6: TR	5	5	Set 12: TR	50	50
Weight/AR			Weight/AR		

Phase 3, Day 4: Cardio, Upper and Lower Abdominals, and Cardio Plus

Date:
Day _____ of 21

A.M. Cardio (30 minutes) ❑
P.M. Cardio (30 minutes) ❑

EXERCISE	SET 1: TR	AR	SET 2: TR	AR	SET 3: TR	AR	SET 4: TR	AR
A.M.: Abdominal Crunches	25		25		25			
A.M.: Lying Leg Raises	25		25		25			
P.M. PLUS: Twists	75/side							

Phase 3, Day 5: Legs and Shoulders

DAY 5

Date:
Day _____ of 21

A.M. Cardio (30 minutes) ❑

	EXERCISE 1	EXERCISE 2		EXERCISE 1	EXERCISE 2
	Squats	Dumbbell Shoulder Press		Squats	Dumbbell Shoulder Press
Set 1: TR	50	50	Set 7: TR	5	5
Weight/AR			Weight/AR		
Set 2: TR	40	40	Set 8: TR	10	10
Weight/AR			Weight/AR		
Set 3: TR	30	30	Set 9: TR	20	20
Weight/AR			Weight/AR		
Set 4: TR	20	20	Set 10: TR	30	30
Weight/AR			Weight/AR		
Set 5: TR	10	10	Set 11: TR	40	40
Weight/AR			Weight/AR		
Set 6: TR	5	5	Set 12: TR	50	50
Weight/AR			Weight/AR		

Phase 3, Day 6: Cardio and Cardio Plus

DAY 6

Date:
Day _____ of 21

A.M. Cardio (30 minutes) ❑
P.M. Cardio (30 minutes) ❑

EXERCISE	SET 1: TR	AR	SET 2: TR	AR	SET 3: TR	AR	SET 4: TR	AR
P.M. PLUS: Twists	75/ side							

Phase 3, Day 7: Cardio and Cardio Plus

DAY 7

Date:
Day _____ of 21

A.M. Cardio (30 minutes) ❑
P.M. Cardio (30 minutes) ❑

EXERCISE	SET 1: TR	AR	SET 2: TR	AR	SET 3: TR	AR	SET 4: TR	AR
P.M. PLUS: Twists	75/ side							

NOTES

_____
_____
_____
_____
_____

Key: TR=Target Reps; AR=Actual Reps

RESOURCES

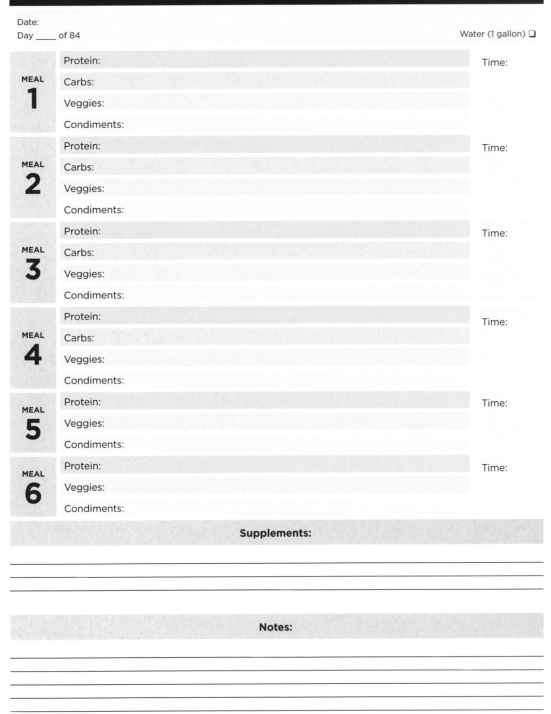

BODY BY DESIGN DAILY NUTRITION TRACKER

Date:
Day _____ of 84

Water (1 gallon) ❑

MEAL 1
Protein:
Carbs:
Veggies:
Condiments:
Time:

MEAL 2
Protein:
Carbs:
Veggies:
Condiments:
Time:

MEAL 3
Protein:
Carbs:
Veggies:
Condiments:
Time:

MEAL 4
Protein:
Carbs:
Veggies:
Condiments:
Time:

MEAL 5
Protein:
Veggies:
Condiments:
Time:

MEAL 6
Protein:
Veggies:
Condiments:
Time:

Supplements:

Notes:

BODY BY DESIGN RECIPES

All recipes here are for one serving, except for the Asian Tuna Patties, which serve four and are perfect for cooking in bulk or to share with friends and family. The amount recommended for chicken, fish, and beef will vary slightly based on the size of your palm, the recommended serving size per meal. The ounces listed represent approximate amounts.

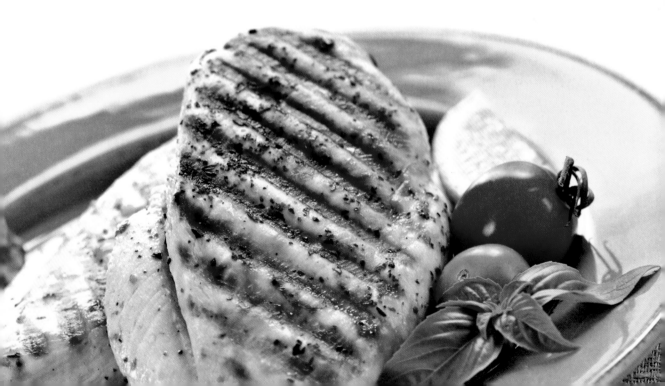

ULTRA OATMEAL

³/₄ cup oatmeal, uncooked

1–2 scoops chocolate protein powder

A few drops mint extract (optional)

Cook the oatmeal in water (as instructed on packaging) and pour into a bowl. Add the protein powder and mix. Turn your chocolate oatmeal into a chocolate mint treat by adding a few drops of mint extract to taste; stir and enjoy.

GROUND TURKEY OMELET

3 ounces ground turkey

½ cup sliced green peppers

½ cup chopped mushrooms

½ clove garlic, chopped

5 egg whites

1 tablespoon salsa

Nonstick cooking spray

In a medium nonstick skillet, sauté the turkey, green peppers, mushrooms, and garlic in cooking spray. In a mixing bowl, whisk the egg whites. Add the egg whites to a second nonstick pan and cook until nearly done. Scoop the turkey mixture onto half of the eggs, folding in half to form an omelet. Add salsa to taste.

VANILLA AND CINNAMON PROTEIN OATMEAL PANCAKES

³/₄ cup oatmeal

4 egg whites

1 scoop vanilla protein powder

Cinnamon (to taste)

1 tablespoon sugar-free syrup

Nonstick cooking spray

Mix the oatmeal, egg whites, and protein powder in a bowl. If additional liquid is needed to mix properly, add a little water and stir until you have a smooth consistency. Spray a frying pan with a nonstick cooking spray, such as Pam, then portion out the mix into pancakes (one or two depending on the size of your pan); cook until brown and firm. Transfer to a plate and add cinnamon and sugar-free syrup to taste.

TUNA OAT PATTIES

1 can tuna, packed in water
¾ cup rolled oats*
2 egg whites, whisked
⅛ cup chopped onion
½ clove garlic, minced
1 tablespoon taco powder
Nonstick cooking spray

Combine the tuna, oats, and whisked egg whites. Stir in the onion, garlic, and taco powder. Mix together and form into patties. Spray a skillet with nonstick cooking spray, place the patties in a skillet, and cook 4 to 5 minutes per side, or until browned.

ASIAN TUNA PATTIES

Four 5-ounce cans tuna, packaged in water
One 16-ounce can garbanzo beans (chickpeas)
5 egg whites
1 onion, finely chopped
1½ tablespoons minced fresh ginger
2 tablespoons low-calorie Dijon mustard
2 tablespoons low-sodium soy sauce
1 teaspoon black pepper
Nonstick cooking spray

In a large mixing bowl, mash the tuna and beans together and then add the rest of the ingredients; mix well. Shape into patties with your hands, making sure that they are tight and firmly packed. Place in a skillet sprayed with nonstick cooking spray. Cook over medium to high heat until lightly browned on the outside.

TORTILLA WRAP

6–8 ounces skinless chicken breast or
   fish fillets
1 cup sliced green or red bell peppers
1 whole wheat tortilla
1 tablespoon salsa

Grill the chicken breast or fish fillets and peppers until lightly charred. Slice the chicken or fish and add with the peppers to the tortilla; top with salsa. Roll up the tortilla and eat—this is great hot or cold. (These are perfect for wrapping up and putting into your food containers for lunch the next day.)

BROILED FISH DIJON

1 tablespoon low-calorie Dijon mustard
½ clove garlic, chopped
6–8 ounces tilapia
1½ pounds small zucchini, cut lengthwise
   into halves
2 slices lemon for juice
Paprika to taste

Mix the mustard and garlic together in a bowl and set aside. In a large baking pan, arrange the fish and zucchini in a single layer. Drizzle with lemon juice. Broil on the top broiler rack for 5 minutes. Turn the fish over and spread

*If you happen to be eating this at a time of the day when your carb intake should be low (after 3 P.M.), replace the rolled oats with finely chopped vegetables.

with the mustard/garlic mixture. Return to the broiler for another 5 minutes, or until the zucchini is lightly browned and the fish is cooked. Sprinkle with paprika to taste.

SALMON STEAKS WITH GINGER

1 tablespoon soy sauce

1/4 teaspoon garlic powder

1 teaspoon fresh ginger, minced

6–8 ounces salmon steak

2 slices lime for juice

Combine the first three ingredients in a bowl and set aside. Heat a skillet over medium to high heat. Add the salmon and cook for about 5 minutes or until browned on one side. Turn and cook for another 4 to 5 minutes, until the salmon flakes easily when tested with a fork. Drizzle with lime juice.

POACHED CHICKEN SALAD

6–8 ounces chicken breast, skinless

1/2 cup water

1 tablespoon dried cilantro

1 tablespoon dried cumin

1 tablespoon dried turmeric

1/4 iceberg lettuce head, chopped

1/4 cucumber, chopped

1 tomato, chopped

2 spring onions, chopped

1 tablespoon lemon juice

Cut the chicken into small pieces and place in a frying pan. Add the water, cilantro, and turmeric and poach for 20 minutes, stirring occasionally. While the chicken is cooking, mix the remaining ingredients except for the lemon juice in a large salad bowl. Drain the chicken and serve it with the salad, finishing with lemon juice to taste.

STEAK AND VEGETABLE STIR-FRY

6–7 ounces sirloin steak

1 cup chopped broccoli

1 cup chopped cauliflower

1 cup sliced mushrooms

1 garlic clove, minced

1 tablespoon Tabasco

Cut the steak into thin slices and place in a frying pan. Stir-fry for about 2 to 3 minutes. Add the vegetables and stir-fry until cooked through. Add the Tabasco sauce and serve.

If you are eating this within your first four meals of the day, you can enjoy it with 3/4 cup cooked brown rice.

ACKNOWLEDGMENTS

A work of this size and scope does not come easily, which is why I wish to thank some important individuals who have made *The Bodybuilding.com Guide to Your Best Body* possible.

First and foremost, my love pours out to my wife, who was patient with me when early mornings and late evenings were necessities in order to make the book a finished product. Thank you for providing me with an endless amount of Tupperware containers filled with wholesome energy to eat and process—your support gave me the power to focus on the task at hand. You are beautiful in every way, Marika.

To my family for teaching me early on that a solid work ethic and trust in my intuition would eventually provide me with the confidence to consistently evolve, mentally and physically.

I cannot express enough how thankful I am to my writer, Gretchen Lees, who spent countless hours extracting my life, beliefs, and passion and turning them into an approachable, sensible, and easy-to-understand work of art that is *The Bodybuilding.com Guide to Your Best Body.* Your talent is incredible.

Stephen Hanselman is a literary agent I could only dream of having—and my dreams came true. Stephen, you told me that this wasn't just a book;

this was an event, and how right you were. It has been the event of my lifetime, and I hope it will be so for millions of others. Your expertise in marketing, editing, public relations, and finding the right publishing partner—even if it meant sprinting the snowy streets of New York—has been first class all around for us at Bodybuilding.com.

To the entire team at Simon & Schuster: you have made this book such a fun and pleasurable experience. We knew as soon as we met that this was going to be a great partnership. I would personally like to thank senior editor Michelle Howry for keeping me organized, preparing me well in advance, and for providing a constant supply of positive energy throughout the entire process. David Falk, as associate publisher, you have done an amazing job of keeping the lines of communication open and helping us share the amazing BodySpace stories with millions of others who can now change their own lives.

As the CEO of Bodybuilding.com, Ryan De-Luca, you make my journey to work a daily dream come true. Words cannot express the gratitude I have to you for allowing me to help millions of people achieve their health, fitness, and appearance goals. You continually prove that you are a dedicated father, husband, and friend, and for that, you will continually have my loyalty. My deepest thanks to you and Jeremy DeLuca for creating such an amazing culture at Bodybuilding.com—you have improved, changed, and saved so many people's quality of life one person at a time, including mine.

And special thanks to photographer Isaac Hinds and model Jacqueline Kay for waking up in the early hours to get the shoot done in one day, and for working hard to make our exercise images come to life.

The soul of this book is about the amazing profiles featured on BodySpace: without you there would be no *The Bodybuilding.com Guide to Your Best Body*. You are the hub of inspiration and viral strength that continues to help millions of people every day. You inspire me, and the BodySpace community, to live healthier lives for friends, family, and coworkers. You are the strength in numbers—continue to lift the world to new heights!

INDEX

PHOTO CREDITS

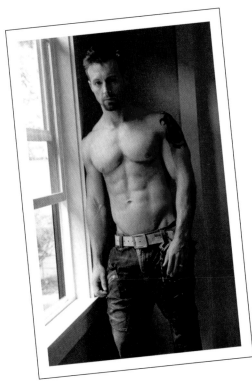

About KRIS GETHIN

KRIS GETHIN is a lifetime natural, drug-free athlete with a background in international health and sports therapy. Since 2005, he has been editor in chief of Bodybuilding.com. His work has also appeared in *Muscle & Fitness, Flex, Iron Man, Musclemag, Body Fitness,* and other publications. With experience as a personal trainer, owner of a fitness center, and bodybuilding writer and photographer, he has dedicated his life to helping promote a healthful and fit lifestyle. Kris still trains thousands daily through video coaching at Bodybuilding.com and is an exclusive fitness coach to several top athletes. He lives in Boise, Idaho, with his wife, Marika.